THE HEALING FACTOR

OPTIMA

THE HEALING FACTOR

A GUIDE TO POSITIVE LIVING

H.E. STANTON

To my family, Valerie, Peter and Lynda, for their good-humoured support and refusal to let me take myself too seriously.

An OPTIMA book

© H.E. Stanton 1981

First published in Australia in 1981 by
Fontana Books
This edition published in 1988 by
Macdonald Optima, a division of
Macdonald & Co. (Publishers) Ltd

A member of Pergamon MCC Publishing Corporation plc

All rights reserved

No part of this publication may be reproduced,
stored in a retrieval system, or transmitted,
in any form or by any means without the prior
permission in writing of the publisher, nor be
otherwise circulated in any form of binding or
cover other than that in which it is published
and without a similar condition including this
condition being imposed on the subsequent
purchaser.

British Library Cataloguing in Publication Data
Stanton, Harry
   The healing factor.
   1. Therapeutic systems
   I. Title
   615.5   R733

0 356 15194 8

Macdonald & Co. (Publishers) Ltd
3rd Floor
Greater London House
Hampstead Road
London NW1 7QX

Photoset in Parliament
Made and printed in Great Britain by
The Guernsey Press Co. Ltd., Guernsey, Channel Islands.

Contents

Preface   10
Acknowledgments   11

PART 1   MEDICINE AND YOU

1. **Medicine—orthodox and unorthodox**   15
   A personal example   15
   Facts and theories   16
   How to look after your health   17
   An example of self-healing   20
   Iatrogenic illness   21
   Natural therapy   24
2. **Taking responsibility for your own health**   27
   Health habits   27
   You create your state of health   29
   Listening to your body   33
   Effective use of your doctor   35
   Your imaginary doctor   39

PART 2   HEALING SYSTEMS

3. **Homoeopathy as a healing system**   45
   Homoeopathy in action   45
   What is homoeopathy?   46
   Homoeopathic prescribing   49
   Potency and dosage   52
   Theories and theories   53

4. **Homoeopathic first aid** 56
    The 'great' remedies 56
    Arnica 56
    Calendula 58
    Urtica urens 59
    Ledum 60
    Nux vomica 60
    Sulphur 61
    Gelsemium 61
    Arsenicum album 63
    Aconite 64
    Bryonia 65
    Rhus toxicodendron 65
    Some other useful remedies 66
    General indicators 70

5. **Bach flower remedies** 72
    Bach's theory of disease 72
    Preparation of the remedies 75
    Dosage 76
    Use of the remedies 77
    Description of the remedies 79
    Some final comments 84

6. **Schuessler's biochemic cell salts and your health** 87
    The Schuessler theory 87
    The twelve cell salts and their uses 88
    Self-treatment of cell salt deficiencies 93
    General principles of self-prescription 95
    Dosage 96
    Food: Mineral salts in their natural form 97
    An overabundance of riches 98

7. **Dowsing for improved health** 99
    The pendulum 99
    Your belief system 101
    Some pendulum exercises 103
    Psychological interference 106

The pendulum and choosing a remedy 108
The concept of harmony 110
Advanced pendulum diagnosis 111
Hand and foot charts 113
Dowsing your vitamins 115
Using charts as an aid to diagnosis 116
Two final ideas 118

8. **Healing through finger pressure** 120
Pressure point therapy 120
Important Acupressure Points 122
Reflex therapy 127
Zone therapy 129
Some specific applications of zone therapy 138

PART 3 DEVELOPING A HEALTHY LIFESTYLE

9. **Nutritional health** 145
The importance of nutrition 145
The principles of good nutrition 147
Food supplements 149
Importance of good eating habits 150
Foods of special value 153
Juices—vegetable and fruit 156
Sprouts 158

10. **Weight control** 159
The problem of overweight 159
Some suggestions on weight control 162
Fasting 164
A plan for gradual weight loss 166

11. **Exercising to improve your health** 170
Being sensible about exercise 170
The safest forms of exercise 172
Exercise and its benefits 175
Setting your exercise goals 178
Pulse rate theory 180

Stretching the body   183
Yoga   184
Isometrics are useful too   184
Exercise as a way of life   185
Some precautions   186

12. **The breath of life**   188
Healthy breathing   188
Breathing for energy   191
Breathing for relaxation   193
Breathing and healing   197
Rhythmic breathing   199
Yogic healing   201

PART 4   THE POWER OF THE MIND

13. **Using your mind to promote good health**   205
Mind and body   205
The power of suggestion   210
Using self-hypnosis to enhance the power of suggestion   212
The problems of stress   219
The relief of stress   219
Controlling pain   222
Using the mind to control weight   224

14. **The healing of faith**   226
Orthodox medicine—from faith to technology   226
Religious faith   230
Increasing your faith through combating fear   233
The healing of bad memories   235
The laying-on of hands   236

PART 5   NATURAL REMEDIES

15. A potpourri of ideas 243
   Water as a healing agent 243
   The treatment of the eyes 247
   Energy and vitality 249
   Insomnia 250
   Ionization of the air 251
   Longevity and stress 253
   Arthritis 255
   Vitamin C 256
   Muscle and leg problems 257
   Digestive problems 258
   A final word 260

   Bibliography 262

   Index 265

Preface

This book is not intended as an attack upon the medical profession which has done much to improve the standard of health in our society. Rather, it takes the view that orthodox Western medicine is only *one* method of health care. Other methods do exist, and it is possible for people to use these methods to take more responsibility for their own health.

In writing this book I make no claim to possession of a special expertise except, perhaps, in the discussion of mental healing. My experience as a psychologist has been of value here. Otherwise, I write as a layman with considerable personal experience in the methods I describe. They have helped me and many, many others to improved health and my hope is they may do the same for you.

Acknowledgments

The ideas outlined in this book come from many sources. Some of these I have referred to specifically in the text. Others remain unacknowledged because I no longer know from whence they came.

I give special thanks to Linda Hornsey and Tony Adams for the part they played in helping me improve on early drafts of the book, and to Angela Brooks for her assistance in the typing of the manuscript.

Part 1
Medicine and You

1. Medicine—Orthodox and Unorthodox

A PERSONAL EXAMPLE

My interest in 'unorthodox' forms of healing began many years ago after I returned from an interstate holiday with a sinus infection. A minor irritation at first, it quickly developed into a serious impairment of my health. I was treated by an orthodox medical practitioner who gave me the usual tests and prescribed the usual drugs and nasal sprays. After more than a year of experiencing the drowsy side effects of antihistamines and the discomfort of the 'bounce-back' effect of nasal sprays, I was told that I'd just have to live with the problem. None of the treatments to which I had been exposed had alleviated the sinus trouble, and no further orthodox treatment was offered.

Being unwilling to live in a state of inferior health, I cast around for avenues other than orthodox medicine which might offer some prospect for a cure. A friend told me about a naturopath who had, over a period of many years, helped his family to attain improved health. After this gentleman examined me, he suggested I warm a bottle of castor oil and place an eye dropper full into each nostril, night and morning. This really sounded peculiar, but I felt I had nothing to lose. Medical treatment had proven quite useless. In fact, I'd often felt worse as a result of the drugs I had been given. Accordingly, I tried the castor oil treatment. After three days, no discomfort remained. I continued for a further three days during which period I experienced none of the previous symptoms of my sinus infection. Since that time, I have had occasional recurrences of the problem, but repetition of the castor oil treatment has seen its immediate disappearance.

This experience, which has been repeated on other occasions with differing minor illnesses, and which has been frequently confirmed by the experience of friends and acquaintants, has made me rather sceptical in accepting at face value the doctor's pronouncement: 'There's nothing more we can do about it. You'll just have to learn to put up with it.' This is not necessarily the last word. Alternatives are available and thousands of people have been cured by methods the medical profession would regard as 'unorthodox' and somehow 'disreputable'.

FACTS AND THEORIES

However, it seems to me that the test of the value of a treatment is not really whether it is accepted as 'orthodox' or 'respectable', but whether it works. Each of us needs to find the things that promote his or her own healing. Everything we believe is a theory, and the only thing our theory has to commend it is whether it works or not. Does it help us to get well and to maintain a state of good health? If it does, for us it is a good theory, a useful guide to how we should behave. If it doesn't, we need to reject it, no matter how many 'experts' tell us it is best for us, and find an alternative approach that makes us feel better.

Orthodox medicine is a theory of health care. Often it has been right. Often it has been wrong. Ivan Illich in *Medical Nemesis*, has documented that virtually every important medical discovery of the last fifty years has, initially, been strenuously opposed by the medical establishment. So orthodox medicine is not infallible. It is not *the* way to health — it is *a* way. The practices of orthodox medicine, though they have taken on something of the status of a dogma, do not necessarily embody *the* truth, enshrined in tablets of stone. It is just a theory which we need to try out for ourselves. The test of its validity for each of us is whether it makes us feel better. Does orthodox medical treatment for a particular ailment improve our health? Other forms of healing might well be approached in the same way.

Several decades ago, a psychologist, Maier, cynically formulated a law which stated that 'if facts do not conform to the theory they must be disposed of'. This is what Illich, in the book referred to earlier, accuses the medical establishment of doing. Where new developments don't fit into the accepted traditional framework, they are rejected. As Russell wrote in his *Report on Radionics*:

> Abrams' shabby treatment by his professional colleagues was no different, of course, from that suffered by Lister, Pasteur, and other great pioneers of the past. In fact, this kind of thing is so common in the history of medicine that a cynic might observe that to be the target of the professional opprobrium is sometimes a certificate of unusual accomplishment . . . Contempt prior to investigation has relegated to oblivion many important truths.

Possibly such statements are overly harsh, but there is a strong tendency to deny the existence of facts which do not match the prevalent orthodox theories. Homoeopathy, which will be discussed later in this book, is a case in point. Margery Blackie, former physician to Queen Elizabeth, has demonstrated over many years the tremendous value of giving patients *Arnica* before and after surgery. Yet, despite the evidence accumulated over thousands of cases, orthodox medicine makes no use of this information. Homoeopathy is a theory which works, and has worked for over 150 years. It is a method which admirably illustrates the basic tenet of healing expounded by the father of medicine, the Greek physician Hippocrates, when he said: 'First, do no harm'. He understood full well that the healing process is part of man, and can be damaged by misguided interventions into nature's workings. Unlike modern drugs, homoeopathic remedies are virtually free from side-effects so, if they do not effect a cure, they do no harm. For many people, it is a theory which works because it brings healing without danger.

HOW TO LOOK AFTER YOUR HEALTH

If orthodox medicine can be seen as *one* way of healing rather than *the* way, how can we best protect our health? That is what this book is all about and, despite my earlier criticism of the inflexibility of some orthodox medical thinking, I would not wish to deny the value of the doctor. Rather, it is a matter of where he fits into our personal health maintenance programme.

Referring back to the example with which the book opened, the pattern was this. Initially I tried to prevent illness through proper nutrition, exercise, and a style of life based on the Socratic dictum of moderation in all things. Despite this preventive action, I contracted a sinus infection. Accordingly I went to a doctor, the normal procedure in our society. When I found his treatment to be ineffective, I sought further specialist medical advice. The result was the same. Because I was unwilling to accept that nothing further could be done, and because I was displeased with the medically prescribed drugs which had increased my discomfort, I sought help from another healing agency. Thus I consulted orthodox medical opinion first, moving into the unorthodox area only when the former had failed me.

An alternative way of handling the situation might have been to attempt unorthodox healing first, before a doctor was approached. This is not as radical a suggestion as it sounds, for most of the visits to physicians are made by patients who lack either the will or the knowledge—or both—to take responsibility for their own minor discomforts. Slight stomach upsets, nervousness, and the occasional headache do not really require highly skilled medical treatment. Initially, these ailments might well be treated by the patient himself, using some of the methods outlined in later chapters. This first step approach could involve pressure point therapy, mental healing, dietary change, or the use of homoeopathy. However, should such methods prove unsuccessful, or should the situation be one of serious illness, the doctor's special skills could be sought. Really it is a matter of the patient taking more responsibility for his own health instead of abdicating totally in favour of a medical 'expert' who is expected to banish illness through the magic of his prescription form.

Hopefully, this book will provide some of the knowledge

necessary for the creation of a more equitable balance between the health care 'experts' and the patient. If we can accept the traditional assumption that the body always seeks to heal itself, therapy, whether it be drugs, homoeopathy, faith, or anything else, serves only to establish the conditions under which the natural healing process thrives. There are times when only a doctor can provide such conditions. However, there are many occasions when a different approach to healing can be equally or more effective, helping to prevent illness and often curing chronic complaints which have resisted the best efforts of orthodox medicine.

Often, these more naturalistic methods are seen as alternatives. Sometimes they are. More commonly, and perhaps more usefully, they may be viewed as adjuncts to orthodox treatment, as a supportive, complementary programme to be used in combination with other therapies. This is the challenge really, how to blend the knowledge and services provided by orthodox medicine with the insight of unorthodox healers to maintain a healthy lifestyle in which illness will be prevented before it occurs.

Such an ideal state is often referred to as holistic health. This concept has as its goal positive well-being in which the individual is vibrantly alive, energetic, self-assured, and free from destructive health habits such as smoking, excessive alcohol intake and overeating. The person who enjoys holistic health is not simply free from obvious illness, which is the usual medical description. The orthodox doctor considers healthy a person whose diagnostic tests reveal no symptoms outside the normal range. Yet this individual might take no exercise, eat a sugar-laden diet, smoke heavily, and impress all who meet him as miserable, inhibited and emotionally repressed. Orthodox medicine looks at symptoms, whereas the unorthodox practitioners see health or illness as related to the whole body function. Disease is not, to them, an isolated symptom or symptoms, but a malfunction of the entire person.

Mind, then, as well as body, is important, for our thoughts and feelings tend to be reflected in our physical condition. When the orthodox medical model concentrates upon pathology and illness, we are encouraged to think along these lines, and so our bodies reflect the symptoms we hear so much about. However, when a model of health is used which concentrates upon wellness rather than upon absence of disease, our thoughts are guided into different channels, ones likely to produce improved physical well being. Hans Selye, in *Stress Without Distress*, has suggested that negative emotions produce chemical changes in the body which are injurious to our health. That is, through the way we think, we can make our bodies ill. If our minds can do this, wouldn't it seem to follow that through the agency of positive emotions they can also make our bodies well? Perhaps love, laughter, faith and hope might have more therapeutic value than we give them credit for. Such eminent physicians as Paracelsus, Holmes, and Osler have gone on record as saying that the history of medication is far more the history of the placebo effort (positive expectancy) than of intrinsically valuable and relevant drugs. Norman Cousins certainly found this to be true.

AN EXAMPLE OF SELF-HEALING

In 1964, this famous American man of letters, while on a visit to Russia, contracted a disease of his connective tissues. Pain was constant, and since the disease was degenerative, Cousins was given only a 1 in 500 chance of surviving. He has written about his illness, providing a graphic description of one man's reaction to the experience of hospitalization:

> I had a fast growing conviction that a hospital was no place for a person who was seriously ill. The surprising lack of respect for basic sanitation, the rapidity with which *staphylococci* and other pathogenic organisms can run through an entire hospital, the extensive and sometimes promiscuous use of X-ray equipment, and the seemingly indiscriminate administration of tranquilizers and powerful painkillers more for the convenience of hospital staff in managing patients than for therapeutic needs ... perhaps the hospital's most serious failure was in the area of nutrition.

Cousins, faced with the virtual certainty of his death, took over his own treatment in partnership with a doctor who supported his decision to heal himself. Feeling it was unreasonable to expect positive chemical changes to take place while his body was being saturated with painkilling medications, Cousins stopped his daily intake of twenty-six aspirins and twelve phenylbutazone tablets. He replaced them with massive doses of intravenous Vitamin C (ascorbic acid), which has been found useful in combating a wide range of illness, though it is still virtually ignored in hospitals and by doctors generally.

To combat his constant pain, now unrelieved by painkillers, Cousins worked on the principle that replacing the negative emotions he had been experiencing with positive emotions might be beneficial. In particular, he embarked on a programme of laughter, watching filmed episodes of 'Candid Camera' at regular intervals. The result, in Cousins' words: 'Ten minutes of genuine belly laughter had an anaesthetic effect and would give at least two hours of pain-free sleep.'

This self-prescribed treatment of Vitamin C and laughter, together with his removal from hospital to a specially set up hotel suite, transformed Cousins from a dying, pain-wracked man to one who is, today, almost fully functional. He plays golf and tennis, rides horses, and is able to live actively in virtually all respects.

There is a message here for all of us who, when we fall ill, wish to promote as rapid a recovery as possible. Cousins was fortunate in having a doctor who encouraged him to believe he was a respected partner in the restoration of health. They had a partnership in which the doctor supported Cousins' efforts to heal himself, accepting his view that the orthodox hospital treatment was ineffective. Many of us are not so fortunate, and though the drug therapy prescribed by our physicians may be helpful, and often is, it can also be very damaging.

IATROGENIC ILLNESS

Cousins' experience points up the dangers of orthodox medicine with its reliance on drug therapy. Many critics of our system of health care have drawn attention to the tendency of modern medicine to overmedicate its patients. Something like one-quarter of the admissions to hospitals today, both in Australia and other Western countries, are attributed to iatrogenic illness. Iatrogenic illness is produced by drugs, either those prescribed by the doctor or those self-prescribed. This is understandable because modern medicine, rather than being cure oriented, is basically a system of symptom suppression. Unfortunately, drugs prescribed to suppress one symptom often create another through side-effects.

Although orthodox medicine has been most effective in preserving life and preventing suffering through antibiotics, vaccines, life support systems, and surgical techniques, the other side of the coin is that adverse drug reactions have become one of the major causes of death. It ranks, in the United States, as the eleventh most deadly killer, claiming approximately 30 000 lives annually. In Great Britain, it has been estimated that every day, half the adults and one third of the children take some form of medication. In France, 30 per cent of illness has been blamed on drug abuse. Professor Higuchi, Professor of Pharmaceutical Chemistry at the University of Kansas, has claimed that ninety per cent of drugs administered are unnecessary, their widespread use promoting illness rather than health.

Our bodies normally operate on a self-regulating basis, producing internally all the chemicals necessary for effective functioning. Therefore, the tendency to use drugs for even the most minor complaint serves only to disturb this desirable self-regulation. As Dr Andrew Malleson puts it in his book *Need Your Doctor Be Useless?*:

> Most of the standard treatments prescribed in general practice for minor physical illnesses not only confound the principles of scientific medicine, but they are even contrary to common sense. They are just silly. The therapeutic attack is delivered not against the cause of the disease, but against the symptoms that the disease causes, and these symptoms are often the body's defence mechanisms against the disease causing agent. Recovery takes place, not because of, but in spite of treatment.

Doctors claim to protect the public against 'charlatan' healers who, at best, achieve nothing for a patient and, at worst, leave him sicker than he was before. Yet surely this same charge could be levelled against orthodox medicine in the illness and death it produces through over-medication. As Dr Donald Norfolk has pointed out in his book, the *Habits of Health*, 'for every five people hooked on heroin, marijuana and LSD, there are 1200 addicted to medically prescribed sedatives'. Obviously, the plea of Sir William Osler, the great Canadian physician, that doctors should educate the masses not to take drugs has been ignored by modern medicine.

The oath of Hippocrates states that the doctor should administer no poison to his patients, even if requested to do so. Yet it is alleged that one patient of every four who die in hospitals is killed by drugs. Something is obviously wrong. In the *Healing Mind*, Dr Oyle comments on this situation, claiming that physicians are unfamiliar with the dangers of the new drugs which they prescribe so freely. Voices such as his, however, are lost against the propaganda of the medical and pharmaceutical industries in their frequent announcements of sensational new developments. The sceptics point out, of course, that should these new developments represent real progress, most people should now be in excellent health with the sick as an exception. Yet, it would seem that today we have an increasing number of people in bad health with more and more new hospitals being built.

Drug therapy is popular among doctors because it is a convenient way of handling large numbers of patients quickly. The patients, too, are at fault for they normally feel 'cheated' if they do not emerge clutching a prescription. Conditioned to believe that drugs are *the* answer, patients put pressure on doctors to fulfil this expectation. So the prescription is a quick way both to satisfy the patient and to permit doctors to feel they have done something useful.

Despite the pressure they put on doctors to prescribe drugs, most patients do not know what drugs they are taking. Surveys quoted by Graedon in *The People's Pharmacy* suggest that patients are unable to identify sixty per cent of the medicines they take and that two-thirds of patients believe the drugs they take are completely safe. Writing as a pharmacist, Graedon believes there is no such thing as a safe drug. Successful treatment, in his opinion, is a careful balance between the beneficial and harmful effects, hopefully weighed in favour of the former. Unfortunately, too often the opposite is the case, with the original illness proving less of a problem than the adverse reaction to treatment.

The victories of orthodox medicine over many diseases have been of tremendous value. However, the history of medicine has not been one of smooth, steady progress. There have been advances, retreats, stagnation, and acrimonious argument between conflicting schools with each one claiming to know the 'one truth'. During this period, doctors have tried remedies which were foolish or, even worse, definitely dangerous. The prevalence of blood letting during the eighteenth century is an example, with blood being taken from patients as a 'cure' for virtually every illness.

In its search for 'the truth', the medical profession has rejected much that is useless and dangerous. Unfortunately, it has also ignored, attacked or discarded much that is of positive value. As people come to realize this, the belief is growing that the practitioner of orthodox medicine can lay no claim to having a monopoly of knowledge about healing. Nor can he present himself as the only person qualified to treat the ill. Many age-old healing skills without drugs and without surgery exist, and this book will explore some of these.

It is obvious, then, why more and more people are turning away from orthodox medicine to seek help from the natural therapies. Disenchantment with drug-oriented medicine is rife. People want more control over their own health. With the complicated nature of medicine today, people feel helpless, at the mercy of doctors, for they have no way of knowing whether the treatment they are receiving is necessary or unnecessary, good or bad. Under such conditions, a turning towards the natural therapies is very understandable.

NATURAL THERAPY

Today, many people are coming to the conclusion that the

remedies of nature are the safest and the most suitable for mankind. Animals heal themselves without drugs or surgery, instinctively seeking solitude where they can relax in safety and use nature's medicines found in plants and pure air. Man seems to have lost this instinctive ability to identify what he requires to maintain health and promote healing. He has replaced instinct with a reliance upon chemical substances which, as has been already pointed out, are something of a mixed blessing. The dangers inherent in the use of modern drugs must surely give some support to those who believe that the treatment of disease should be as natural as possible.

Since the days of Hippocrates, and probably well before, health conscious individuals have stressed the value of water, fresh air, exercise, and natural foods in creating a sound constitution likely to resist the inroads of illness. Should sickness occur, the body, made fit through sensible living, will be better able to recover through natural healing processes without recourse to drugs and operations.

This concept is basically that of a life force, or healing power within the body, which works to restore balance and health. Some things such as fresh air, plain diet, massage, and water treatment strengthen the life force. Others, such as smoking, excessive alcohol intake and overeating, weaken it.

This idea of encouraging the life force so the body is better able to resist disease is central to the naturopathic view to healing. This approach differs markedly from that of orthodox medicine with its emphasis upon 'germ theory'. In *How to Get Well*, Paavo Airola has this to say about 'germ theory':

> ... the twentieth century concept of disease is not much different from the primitive voodoo concept. The only difference is that the 'evil spirits' have been replaced with 'evil germs', bacteria or virus, which attack the unfortunate and undeserving man. We believe that disease 'strikes' the unsuspecting and totally innocent bodies. We talk about diseases as being 'caught'. We speak of evil creatures—the germs—as 'going around', attacking every man in their way. The job of the modern medicine man is to kill or drive out the evil intruders, the germ or virus, with the magical medical power from his medicine bottle or injection needle, and thus, save the innocent victim from the vicious attack.

Naturopaths don't share the doctors' germ theory of disease. Germs may exist but whether they actually affect a particular individual will really depend on that person's existing state of health. Whereas the medico uses drugs to defeat the germs, the naturopath attempts to strengthen the body so it will not provide an easy target. It is basically the difference between preventing disease before it can start, and attempting to cure it once it has started. Such prevention is a matter of lifestyle, and the naturopath functions as a teacher, guiding the patient into adoption of a healthier way of life. Germs and viruses may exist, but they are thought of as responses to a lifestyle which is disharmonious with the environment. But no one can force you to change the way you live. That is a personal decision for which you must take responsibility.

You need also to take responsibility for making a choice among the various modes of treatment available to you. After consideration of unorthodox approaches, you may decide they are not for you, that the orthodox medical model satisfies your needs. However, should you believe modern medicine has become overconcerned with a non-curative approach to illness through its emphasis upon the treatment of symptoms, you may wish to choose an alternative. No one else can do this for you. Your choice involves the issue of personal responsibility, a theme to be elaborated in the next chapter.

2. Taking Responsibility for Your Own Health

HEALTH HABITS

As mentioned in the last chapter, most of us have been conditioned to think that a disease is due to germs, bad luck, or malignant fate. If we choose to think in this way, we can disclaim all responsibility for our own health. We are sick because of something 'out there' which does this terrible thing to us. But this is simply not true. Much illness and disease is due to the living habits we choose to adopt, and we will never heal ourselves by taking drugs. Such medication may lead to temporary improvement. Often it doesn't. If the erroneous living habits remain unchanged, the illness inevitably recurs.

There is a growing realization that, if modern disease is primarily a result of lifestyle and the environment, *the only remedy likely to be effective lies in the hands of the individual.* Prevention of illness is basically a matter of transforming your life through the adoption of certain health habits. There is nothing magical about these—nor are they strikingly new or unusual. Rather they are simply common sense principles which have been recognized as conducive to good health for many years:

- three regular meals a day without in-between snaks
- breakfast every day
- moderate weight
- no smoking
- moderate drinking
- seven or eight hours drug-free sleep a night
- moderate regular exercise two or three times a week.

A University of California public health survey of 7000 adults, showed with amazing consistency that people maintaining all seven of these habits enjoyed better health than those with six and that those with six enjoyed better health than those with five. This difference continued right down the line so that people with only one or none of these seven health habits were the unhealthiest of all those who took part in the survey. Such evidence does suggest quite strongly that lifestyle is a crucial factor in sickness and health. If some power could suddenly end the abuse of alcohol, tobacco and cars, more than half the beds in hospitals would suddenly become empty.

Easier said than done. As Dr John Diamond said in *Your Body Doesn't Lie*:

> Early in my internship I realized that most of my patients wanted only to be relieved of any symptoms that were causing them difficulty . . . so that they could go back to the poor health habits they had before. So few seemed to want to change, to be really well . . . I could never get it through to them that their well-being was their own responsibility.

Perhaps I may have more success in this book, for succeeding chapters will set out many ways in which you can prevent illness, improve your general health, and heal yourself should you fall sick. However, until we all recognize that we have to look after ourselves, all the good advice in the world will fall upon deaf ears. The problem is one of motivating people to want to be healthy; to be sufficiently concerned to actually make an effort to change nutritional habits such as avoiding sugar and artificially processed foods; to reduce drug intake, including alcohol, tobacco, and caffeine; and to get adequate exercise and sleep. Improved health will not just happen—we have to make it happen. Responsibility for your health and your body lies not with your medical expert, but with yourself.

Our medical model is at fault here, for it assumes that people are weak and irresponsible, capable only of complete dependence upon an expert, the doctor. Patients are expected to believe that the doctor has all the answers. He will diagnose the problem and provide the cure. For most of us, medicine is considered as our *only* resource in time of illness, and physicians rarely help patients to realize their own power to heal themselves. Unfortunately, orthodox medicine frequently fails to meet these high expectations. It assumes a greater responsibility for the health of its patients than it can discharge. This leads to considerable dissatisfaction on the part of patients.

YOU CREATE YOUR STATE OF HEALTH

The famous psychologist, Carl Jung, claimed that everything that happens to a person is a direct result of that person's thinking, speaking, and actions. That is, the diseases we have are seen as a direct expression of our total life situation, and it might be useful for us to consider whether some illnesses exist because they serve a purpose, because they meet a need we might have. This is akin to saying that we can make ourselves ill.

Greg Balsam did so regularly. Greg is a real person but his name, as are all those used as case study examples in this book, is fictitious. Whenever the pressure of work became too much, he developed a severe cold which incapacitated him for several days. His eyes streamed, his nose ran, he developed a bad cough, and he experienced severe chills. Though these colds occurred several times a year, Greg never realized why he suffered in this way. He did not realize that when we subject our body to severe stress, it reacts self-defensively. This may take the form of acute symptoms such as pain, fever, fatigue, or loss of appetite, which tend to make the patient slow down, reduce food intake and get more rest. If the patient heeds these warning signs he stays home in bed for a couple of days, recuperates, gains relief from the stressful work environment, and recovers.

However, in Greg's case, unless he realizes what is causing his body to develop a cold as a self-defence measure, his situation will not improve. Somehow he needs to reduce the stress of his work and, if unable to do so, might consider changing jobs. This is a more responsible attitude to take than to suppress the pain and fever with drugs, and to keep forcing in food which the body does not want. A change in lifestyle might be the only way in which Greg will get rid of his colds.

It is easy to talk of changing lifestyle habits, of course. Actually doing it may not be quite so easy, probably because of the way we choose to go about it. Usually we work really hard at overcoming bad habits, concentrating all our will power upon telling ourselves we must not continue to behave in a particular way. Don Wheelis, constantly plagued by ill-health, decided to give up cigarettes and alcohol. He focussed on his bad habits, exhorting himself to overcome them, and constantly berating himself for his backsliding. Sometimes he would go without a drink or a cigarette for a week or two, then he'd weaken and find himself smoking and drinking as much as usual. Obviously, for Don, as for most of us, concentrating on giving up a negative habit just doesn't work.

An alternative approach is to adopt a positive habit. This might be meditation or jogging, for example, two activities which serve to calm the mind, promote relaxation, and, incidentally, reduce the need for 'relaxants' such as tobacco and alcohol. Often these drugs simply drop out of a person's life as he reduces stress through increased fitness and improved nutrition. When Don started breathing hard during exercise three or four times a week, reduced his sugar and salt intake, and drifted into the healing silence engendered by relaxation and meditation for a short period each day, his health improved dramatically. Through concentration on positive habits, Don enhanced his life, letting go the negative habits of smoking and drinking almost incidentally. As Hippocrates put it: 'When one has fallen sick we must change our way of living, for it is evident that the one we followed was erroneous wholly or in great part.'

Unfortunately, we are often encouraged to adopt a way of living which is actually detrimental. For example, the world of advertising is constantly exhorting us to take antacids for every minor stomach upset. It also promotes laxatives, pain relievers, nasal decongestants, and a multitude of other preparations which, taken indiscriminately, may not only be relatively ineffective in giving us the relief we seek, but can possibly contribute to a worsening of our condition. It is, then, not only the doctors who overprescribe. We do it ourselves, encouraged by the advertising to which we are continually subjected. If we dose ourselves with the many preparations 'pushed' in this way, we may enrich the pharmaceutical companies, but we are unlikely to create the healthier life which is our goal.

This concept of taking responsibility for our own health can be taken too far, of course. It is something of an overstatement to claim that complete responsibility for your health and your body lies not with your doctor but with yourself. There are environmental pressures over which we have no control. Pollution in our cities, for example, is difficult to avoid. Much illness is generated through the working conditions people are forced to endure. The problems with asbestos and lead are well known, as are those with many industrial chemicals which have detrimental effects upon our health. Unfortunately, the people who will prove these chemicals as unsafe are those who, 30 years from now, will have been exposed to them for 10, 20 or 30 years. Sometimes we can avoid these influences, but often we cannot because we simply do not realize the danger to which we are exposed. For many years housewives cooked meals for their families in aluminium utensils, unaware of the adverse effect large and continuous doses can have on the health of some individuals.

Heredity factors, too, are normally beyond our control. Much disease is of this sort and there is little that the individual can do in such cases. Neither can he do anything about the brain damage he may have suffered at birth. However, pregnant women can, at least, be particularly careful about their intake of drugs during the gestation period. The thalidomide tragedy stands as a grim reminder of the damage that can be visited upon unborn babies.

Thus, though we can be responsible for our own health only up to a certain point, most of us can do far more than we are doing. Reverting to the example of the aluminium saucepans, even today such cooking utensils are still used by housewives. Perhaps they remain in ignorance of the danger, or perhaps they simply cannot be bothered changing to an alternative. Apathy in health matters abounds and is probably the main obstacle to improvement in this area. If we can accept the naturopathic view that the main cause of disease is not the bacteria, virus or germ, but the weakened resistance in man caused by health-destroying living habits and physical and emotional stress, the path to improved health is obvious. We need to build up our resistance so the germs are unable to affect us, and later chapters of this book suggest ways in which this might be done.

Medicine and health should not be thought of as meaning the same thing. The components of health include nutrition, the efficient functioning of our physical bodies, and our mental and emotional balance. Drugs and surgery, the tools of orthodox medicine, are of only limited value in facilitating improvement in this area so we cannot delegate to a doctor the responsibility for our well-being. Perhaps we have now reached a stage where further progress in health will be a result of our learning the skills of self-care rather than through the technology of scientific medicine. In this way we promote our own health instead of relying on doctors to repair us when we fall ill. As Anne Wigmore says in *Be Your Own Doctor*:

> How unfortunate it is that we have become dependent upon others to take care of our mental, physical and spiritual duties. When our spiritual leader explains his spiritual beliefs, we gulp them down as gospel. When the psychologist explains the methods our thinking should be geared to, we accept the instructions without questioning. When the physician tells us to take this or that, we accept the suggestions as ultimatums. And when we find ourselves in predicaments, we usually blame others for our difficulties.

First, heal yourself, and you may then act as a model for others, encouraging improved health among your family, friends, acquaintances and colleagues. However, it is useless to preach health improvement if you do not practise it yourself. I remember my reaction to a leading speaker at a conference on heart disease. He came to the rostrum smoking a cigar and carrying at least twenty kilograms excess weight. The previous evening I had seen him consuming copious amounts of alcohol so when he finally staggered off to bed he could hardly see straight. Yet this man spoke about risk factors in heart disease, telling his audience they should eliminate tobacco from their lives, eat moderately, and reduce their alcohol intake. His words said one thing. However, his behaviour said that he did not really believe his own words. I, and many others in the audience, were unable to hear his words, to take them seriously, when the man himself transmitted a different message. Who we are speaks louder than what we say. As you take responsibility for your own health, you not only enhance your own life. You are also likely to enhance the lives of those around you.

LISTENING TO YOUR BODY

To improve your own health it is necessary to become more sensitive to the messages of your body. Often these are very faint, but if detected, they warn you that, unless you make changes in your activities, you are going to become ill. These messages act as signals, suggesting you may need more sleep, a change of diet, or a change of environment to improve your physical condition. Learning to detect these signals enables you to take positive action to restore health and harmony to your life. This is relatively easy to do before illness sets in. It is more difficult to do once you become ill.

Some messages are easy to interpret. If you feel pain, you are being told not to move a certain part of the body because doing so is likely to interfere with the body's healing process, wasting energy which could better be used to aid your recovery. Hoarseness in the throat, loss of voice, is another obvious signal suggesting you're talking too much or too loudly, and perhaps spending too much time in smoke-filled rooms. Indigestion after meals indicates you should be looking more closely at what you are eating, observing whether your discomfort regularly follows after consuming certain foods or drinks.

The body reports its adverse reactions through such

symptoms. These signals often suggest what we should do as far as treatment is concerned. Frequent sneezing involves a loss of fluid—so drinking increased amounts of water is likely to be helpful. A stuffy nose which is making breathing difficult suggests nose drops to decrease swelling, although too frequent use of nose drops may cause a 'bounce-back' effect which aggravates the problem. The sore throat requires a hot water gargle, perhaps with some salt added, to encourage an increased blood flow to the affected area.

Responding to the body's messages helps you avoid illness which usually arrives after you have repeatedly ignored these signals. If, when you had first noticed the roughness in your throat, you had restricted your talking, stopped smoking for a day or two, and increased your fluid intake, your body might well have repaired itself so that no serious problem developed. By heeding the message of your symptoms, you might have taken additional Vitamin C, used hot water and salt gargles, and slowed down a bit, getting extra relaxation and sleep. That is, by taking such early action, you practise a preventive medicine which will drastically reduce the number of visits you need to make to your doctor.

Practitioners of holistic medicine talk of health in terms of being in harmony with your environment. When this harmony is not present, various symptoms appear. Insomnia, for example, is not an ailment but a message to you to get your life into better order. Establish a regular bedtime routine; avoid late evening stimulants, such as coffee; cope with your personal problems; think pleasant thoughts rather than agonize over the worries of the day, and get more exercise.

In contrast to the negative body messages I have been describing, we may receive positive signals. As we bask in a glow of well-being our body is telling us we have been doing something right, something we might well repeat. Perhaps we have eaten a meal which has made us feel good, or maybe we have turned off our worries through relaxing in the sun. Possibly we have been somewhere where we have breathed deeply of pure, fresh air. Whatever it is that has generated this feeling of contentment, heed your body's satisfaction, identify the source of it, and do it again whenever possible. Listening to your body helps you prevent sickness, but despite your vigilance there will be occasions when you fall ill. At such times your doctor can be a valuable health resource—if you use him or her effectively.

EFFECTIVE USE OF YOUR DOCTOR

In his excellent book *How to Be Your Own Doctor (Sometimes)* Dr Keith Schnert sets out valuable guidelines on ways of getting the best from your medico. As a physician himself Schnert's advice is particularly pertinent. He quotes 'Mrs Meek' as an example of how a patient should not act. She is quite passive, totally dependent upon the information a busy physician decides to tell her. She asks no questions in the examination room, partly because she believes the doctor would brook none, and partly because she does not know the appropriate questions to ask. Mrs Meek is a person to whom things are done, someone who submits 'to the divine will'. Patients like Mrs Meek do not question, do not challenge, do not doubt— and often do not get the treatment which is their right.

Schnert provides an alternative model in which the patient develops a partnership with the doctor so that the responsibility for restoring health is a shared one. Your doctor can be of great value to you, but the extent to which he is able to help you depends, to a large extent, on you. You need to communicate with your doctor, and to do so, you would be well advised to begin before your appointment. In the surgery, it is easy to forget to ask about all the little things you wanted to discuss. You tend to concentrate only upon your major complaint, perhaps neglecting to bring out some of the main details even here. To prevent this, write down beforehand on a card the questions you want to ask, and take your list along with you. Perhaps your doctor will take your card and go over the points one at a time with you. His recommendation can then be noted on the reverse side of the card.

What questions should you ask your doctor? Schnert provides a very useful list.

THE ASK-THE-DOCTOR LIST

A Before the visit (complete this part yourself)
1. Why am I going to the doctor? (the main reason) _____
   _____
2. Is there anything else that worries me about my health?
   _____ No
   _____ Yes (please list) _____
3. What do I expect the doctor to do for me today? (in 10 words or less) _____

B During the visit (complete with help of doctor)
1. What is the diagnosis? _____
2. Why did I get it and how can I prevent it next time? ___
   _____
3. Are there any helpful patient education materials available for the condition? (describe) _____
   _____
4. Are there any medicines for me to take?
   _____ No
   _____ Yes (describe) _____
5. Are there any special instructions, concerns, or possible side effects I need to know about the medicine?
   _____ No
   _____ Yes (describe) _____

C After the visit (complete with help of doctor)
1. Am I to return for another visit?
   _____ No
   _____ Yes (when) _____
2. What should I do at home?
   _____ Activity _____
   _____ Treatments _____
   _____ Precautions _____
3. Am I to phone in for lab reports?
   _____ No
   _____ Yes (when)
4. Should I report back to doctor by phone for any reason?
   _____ No
   _____ Yes (when)

The patient eager to take more responsibility for his own health asks many questions. If the doctor doesn't tell you what is wrong with you—ask. What is the problem? Its cause? How can it be prevented from recurring? Should the doctor's explanation be too technical, ask him to explain in words you can understand. In particular, be quite clear about the medication prescribed. What is its name? How often should you take it? When should you take it (before meals, with meals)? Should you take it with water, milk, juice? Is there the possibility of side effects? What should you do if these side effects do appear? Keep a record of any side effects you experience, and tell the doctor about these together with information about any allergies you may have. Also let him know whether you are taking any other drugs.

It is particularly useful to ask whether there are other things you can do besides taking the medication which will assist your recovery. Perhaps an increased fluid intake, bed rest, walking in the fresh air, might be more valuable in helping the body heal itself than the prescribed drug. If you do not feel happy about the prescribed treatment, say so. The doctor may be able to suggest alternative healing methods which are likely to work just as well for you. Should he be unable to suggest a treatment approach which makes you feel good, seek other advice.

You have to trust your doctor. Without faith in his ability to assist the healing process, you can drastically reduce the effectiveness of the treatment he prescribes. Numerous studies exist which indicate that a placebo, an inert medication, will promote healing if prescribed by a doctor in whom the patient believes. The same placebo, prescribed by a doctor in whom the patient has no faith, achieves nothing. When the placebo is replaced by an active drug, one which has a measurable chemical effect, its healing power is greatly enhanced if you trust your physician. If you lack this trust, find another doctor.

So many patients are loathe to do this. They put up with doctors who give the impression of being too busy to see them, who make patients feel as if they have been an imposition, and who make people wait for hours to see them. Doctors sell you a service, and part of this service is to communicate with you so your doubts and fears are eased. If they are not giving you the information you require about your body and its treatment, they are not providing the service for which you are paying them. By not answering your questions and not clearing up your doubts and fears, they are denying you your right of participating as fully as possible in your own healing. Quelling your fears about disease is at least as important as getting a prescription for a drug. If your doctor makes you feel foolish about asking questions, change doctors until you find one with whom you can communicate, one who is willing to let you co-operate in the treatment of your own body.

Try, also, to get a doctor who sees you reasonably promptly. It is not unusual to find yourself waiting at the surgery for an hour, or even longer, despite having made a definite appointment. Sometimes there is an excellent reason why the doctor is running well behind his schedule—an unexpected emergency for example. More commonly, the reason why you have to wait is because more appointments have been made than the doctor can comfortably handle in the time available. No one makes the physician do this. He chooses to do so, overcrowding his schedule month after month, year after year. Why should he do this? Economic benefit would seem to be the only reason, and he will continue to waste your time in this way unless you complain. The unspoken message, according to Samuels and Bennett in the *Well Body Book*, is that your time is less valuable than that of the doctor. No one has the right to 'waste' another person's time in this way, but you allow your medico to do so if you make of him an authority figure, accepting that his time is more important than yours, and being too inhibited to complain.

Let your doctor know that long delays annoy you, and that you do not intend to wait more than a certain time, perhaps half an hour. If you have not been seen within the half hour, leave, letting the receptionist know. It is useful to write the doctor a note explaining your action. Then seek another medical adviser who does not overcrowd his schedule and can see you at the time for which he makes the appointment. Unless patients assert themselves, doctors will continue to treat them as if their time was unimportant. However, if enough of his patients demonstrate they will not tolerate such treatment, a doctor's behaviour is likely to change. Loss of income is a very effective corrective. Doctors need to be questioned and challenged if we are to gain the service for which we pay.

YOUR IMAGINARY DOCTOR

Your doctor can help you if you use him intelligently. So, too, can the imaginary doctor you create in your own mind. Actually, your creation does not have to be a doctor, but can be anyone or anything, person, animal or object, that you can use to assist you in the improvement of your health.

One way of 'meeting' your assistant is to imagine yourself in a pleasant room, relaxed and at ease. This room is a sanctuary for you, for while you are in it nothing can disturb or worry you. You make it perfect—the way you want it to be. Perhaps you relax yourself by taking deep, slow breaths, sending your breath to each part of the body in turn. As your breath reaches say, your left foot, feel it relax and let go. Then send successive breaths to the left ankle, calf muscle, knee, thigh and hip so the entire leg is at ease. Similarly, relax the right leg, stomach lower back, chest, upper back, arms, neck, face and scalp. Actually, as you become used to sending your breaths to relax your body, you can speed up the process, 'letting go' the leg as a whole instead of its separate parts. Of course, there are many other ways of relaxing the body and mind. (Chapters 12 and 13 will outline some of these.)

Once your body is relaxed and your mind calm, you might imagine that you are looking at a door in one wall of your special room. This is a very special door which opens by sliding down into the floor. Your assistant or doctor is behind this door which you control from the chair in which you are sitting. Gradually lower the door, so you can see his or her hair, eyes and face, letting the features emerge spontaneously. Similarly allow the body to emerge slowly, until you have a clear picture in your mind. As your assistant steps into the room you talk with him or her, learning his or her name, and allowing aspects of personality to appear. Just let it happen. Don't try to force it in any way by attempting to pre-select who your helper is to be. Let him, her or it develop spontaneously. Unless your assistant, or assistants, for maybe more than one will appear, come to you on a subconscious level with no interference from your conscious mind, they are unlikely to be of much use to you.

Although the idea of creating an imaginary helper may seem strange, it is nothing new. Many people living in cultures different from our own, such as some American Indian tribes, have invoked a personal spiritual adviser to guide them through life. This entity can be consulted when problems arise, when trustworthy advice is required. As this book is concerned with your health, it seems appropriate to suggest your assistant might well be a doctor who practises orthodox medicine, a naturopath, a faith healer, or anyone else whose healing power you trust. However, as I've described in an earlier book, *The Plus Factor*, your helper can advise you on any matter you choose to discuss so you are free to create anyone or anything your subconscious mind desires.

There are no 'right' imaginary assistants—the one or ones you get are likely to be right for you. Should you create one you don't like, that makes you feel uncomfortable, let it go, wiping your mind clear and repeating the exercise until you have someone or something you can trust to help you. The variety of assistants people create is great, ranging from familiar figures such as parents, religious figures, teachers, through other human beings who are strangers, to non-human forms such as glowing crystals and colours. As you become increasingly comfortable with your helper you will find yourself sharing many problems. Often these will be of a medical nature. Perhaps your helper will diagnose your ailment, suggesting appropriate treatment. At other times you will check out a healing method you would like to use, seeking approval or disapproval. You might imagine your helper actually healing you, applying a special ointment to a skin infection or giving you a healing medicine to cure a stomach upset. As you become increasingly familiar with the possibilities, you will be impressed with the healing that can be generated in this way. And *you* are doing it.

Invocation of an imaginary helper and using your orthodox doctor effectively are part of a general theme, that of taking more responsibility for your own body. When you do so, not only will your health improve but your self-esteem will increase. You will realize that you have resources, previously neglected, which make you a more effective human being. That is a very self-enhancing discovery to make. Another exciting discovery is that systems of medicine exist which you can use on a self-help basis without specialized knowledge. One of these is homoeopathy.

Part 2
Healing Systems

3. Homoeopathy as a Healing System

HOMOEOPATHY IN ACTION

Chris Harrington is a delightful child, three years old and full of high spirits. At least, he used to be. The affliction of severe constipation came as a blight upon his young life and his normally sunny disposition gave way to tears. Medical treatment with laxatives achieved nothing, though it did contribute to very painful episodes when Chris' bowels did move. Naturally his parents were very distressed, and, as the months passed, became increasingly disenchanted with the treatment provided. Seeking an alternative, they were advised to discontinue laxatives and use the homoeopathic remedy, *Bryonia*, which is made from wild hop. Three doses a day initially, then a gradual reduction as Chris' condition improved, proved sufficient to banish the constipation and the pain of the bowel movements.

An exceptional case perhaps? Not at all. Tony Bittern, a hard-driving business man, became increasingly irritable with his wife, children and business associates. Tense, on-edge, nervous, Tony frequently 'exploded' over trivialities. He was advised to take tranquillizers but refused to do so, fearing their side effects would have a detrimental effect upon his work capacity. However, he was willing to use the poison nut, *Nux vomica*, a homoeopathic remedy which has no such side effects. Four doses achieved the desired improvement, restoring Tony's equilibrium and good temper without reduction of his energy and clear thinking.

The use of poison nut in the above example sounds ominous.

Even more so sounds *Tarantula cubensis*, a remedy made from the venom of the Cuban black spider. The bite of this spider will produce an inflamed pimple which develops into an abscess, much like a carbuncle. Yet, the homoeopathic remedy is an excellent treatment for carbuncles and boils.

The same apparent contradiction can be seen in the action of other remedies. A large dose of *Ipecacuanha* causes nausea and vomiting in a healthy individual. A small dose, used in accordance with homoeopathic principles, cures nausea in the dyspeptic individual. Similarly, *Arsenic* given in large doses to a healthy person produces a severe stomach ache, vomiting and diarrhoea, all symptoms of food poisoning. Small doses of the same substance relieve the symptoms of food poisoning.

Belinda Peters had cause to bless the power of a remedy created from another poisonous substance. Her urticaria, an 'allergic' skin reaction, became severe, the itching of the raised red weals which appeared on her body driving her to distraction. Nothing helped, the various ointments and lotions she tried all aggravating the problem rather than giving relief. *Apis*, or honey bee poison, a homoeopathic remedy, provided the answer. Yet, in its natural form, bee venom produces a red, itchy burning oedema, the very symptoms from which Belinda suffered.

Belinda's case, and those of Chris and Tony described earlier, are real, although their names are fictitious. They are typical of the thousands of people who have been helped by homoeopathy, which is perhaps the most successful form of self-help medicine available to the layman. Not everyone will respond with instant, spectacular success to the use of homoeopathic remedies, but the chances are good that most of us can find some measure of relief from our ailments.

WHAT IS HOMOEOPATHY?

Consideration of the examples outlined above give some idea of the basic principles upon which homoeopathy is founded. Perhaps the most obvious of these is the 'law of similars', or like cures like. The symptons which a substance, be it plant, mineral or animal, causes in overdoses, can be removed by the same substance when given in specially prepared, infinitesimal doses. Samuel Hahnemann, the German physician and chemist who founded homoeopathy at the end of the eighteenth century, tested his remedies on the healthy before using them on the sick, and found that the more decreased the amount administered, the greater the effect. This was true even when there remained virtually no trace of the original substance.

This use of infinitesimal doses, called the 'law of potencies', has been the main reason why homoeopathy has not received more widespread acceptance. It is difficult to believe that such minute amounts of a substance, repeatedly diluted, could exert any healing effect. This repeated dilution, together with a process termed succussion, is the means through which the homoeopathic remedy is prepared.

Petroleum, an excellent remedy for travel sickness, can serve as an example. One part of petroleum is mixed with nine parts of a diluting medium, usually distilled water and alcohol. This mixture is then shaken vigorously, usually by mechanical means, the procedure being termed succussion. However, for the person preparing his own medicines, the bottle containing the mixture can be struck against the palm of the hand about 15 times. The medicine is now dubbed 1X. One part of this mixture may again be diluted with nine parts of water and alcohol and succussed. It is now a 2X potency. The process can be continued to create 6X, 12X, 30X or 200X potencies, which are those most commonly used.

An alternative to the decimal scale described above is the centesimal scale, where one part of petroleum would be mixed with 99 parts of water and alcohol to create a 1C potency. One part of this dilution would again be diluted with 99 parts of water and alcohol, and so on. Mathematicians have established that by about the 10C potency, no molecules of the original substance will be left. Therefore, theoretically the remedy should have no healing power—but it does.

So we are faced with a paradox, one which runs through the fabric of our society. We possess this rather peculiar human attribute of ignoring the fact that something works, and concentrating on the lack of a theory or explanation. That is, we ignore the evidence of our eyes because we have no plausible theory to explain why things are happening the way they do. I would suggest that each of us should become our own expert, and try out things for ourselves. Even if you are told a certain healing approach cannot work, try it out for yourself. It may work for you. Conversely, if you do try out a form of healing, be it the latest wonder drug or a natural remedy, and find it doesn't help you, let it go and try something else, no matter how many experts tell you how wonderful it is. Experts are right — sometimes. They are also wrong — frequently. So I would suggest you treat the ideas presented in this book in a very practical way. Try them and see whether they help you. If they do, fine. Keep using them whether anyone has come up with a theory to explain why they work or not. Obviously medical emergencies do not fall into this category. In those cases you require orthodox medical help fast. However, most of our ailments are not medical emergencies, but nagging minor problems, some acute, some chronic. These you can experiment upon, and become an expert in the healing of your own body.

Louise Bellings, for example, has learnt that the common daisy, *Bellis perennis*, makes her life easier, despite the fact that the 12X solution she takes can theoretically have no effect upon her at all. As a garden lover, Louise often spends hours among her vegetables and flowers. Particularly on days when the sun is shining, she overdoes it somewhat, dragging herself inside with an aching back and sore muscles. However, having been told about *Bellis*, the 'gardener's remedy', she immediately takes five drops in a little water. Perhaps she repeats the dose several times over the next few hours until the muscle soreness disappears. And disappear it does. It should not work — yet it does. As I said earlier, trust the evidence of your senses.

Perhaps it is all a placebo effect. Webster's *Dictionary* defines a placebo as 'an inert medication given for its psychological effect especially to satisfy the patient' and as 'something tending to soothe and gratify'. That is, a placebo actually has no power in itself, but achieves a healing effect because the patient believes it has curative power. This may be a possible explanation of the success achieved by homoeopathic remedies, though many very sceptical people have experienced healing, together with babies, animals and plants. It is difficult to accept that an ailing tomato plant, battered by a high wind, can recover dramatically because it 'believes' in the curative power of a few drops of the shock remedy, *Arnica,* placed upon its leaves. Still, stranger things have happened. Whether homoeopathy achieves its healing effect through some power of its own, or through the placebo effect, it does promote healing, and has done so for the best part of 200 years.

Many practising homoeopaths do, however, claim that, as a result of the dilution and succussion preparation procedure, the energy latent in the substance is liberated and increased. Dr Stephenson, for example, in his excellent book, *A Doctor's Guide to Helping Yourself with Homoeopathic Remedies,* suggests that the preparation procedure 'frees up' the healing energies in the medicine. That is, he sees them acting as carriers of energy rather than as chemical drugs, their action being one of helping the patient heal himself. Homoeopathy thus cooperates with our inherent self-healing capacity in a very gentle, safe way, providing a marked contrast with traditional medicine which believes in a chemical onslaught to destroy invading germs. Because of their supportive, gentle action, homoeopathic remedies offer a safe beginning to treatment.

Our error, I believe, is that we turn to drugs and surgery as first alternatives instead of waiting until we have exhausted natural, harmless forms of treatment such as homoeopathy, and the other alternatives discussed in later chapters. Though conventional medical wisdom would suggest such a procedure to be dangerous because of the possible ill-effects of postponing the 'proper' treatment, this would be true for only a very small percentage of the ailments with which we are troubled. In fact, the danger may well be less than that involved in taking the powerful drugs likely to be prescribed for the ailment.

HOMOEOPATHIC PRESCRIBING

It is a theory that homoeopathic remedies act as carriers of energy which restore the harmony of the body through stimulating the organism to heal itself. It may or may not be true. Homoeopaths subscribe, also, to another theory concerning how remedies should be chosen. They see a patient as an individual, as a trilogy of body, mind and spirit, so that treatment must be directed towards the whole person. Thus, the homoeopathic process involves a very detailed initial interview which clarifies the unique way a person exhibits his physical and psychological symptoms. An individualized remedy is then chosen, based upon its ability to create the similar totality of symptoms if a healthy person took it in large quantities. Hahnemann set the pattern for this approach to prescribing, believing that he should treat the patient rather than the disease. The result is that a single remedy is often able to relieve a number of physical, emotional and mental complaints at the same time. *Nux vomica*, mentioned earlier as successful in relieving Tony Bittern's irritability, also 'cured' him of a flatulent stomach, cramps in his feet at night, wakefulness at 3–4 a.m., and his hangovers.

However, considerable time is necessary. The homoeopathic practitioner has to learn all he can about his patient's temperament, constitution, background and needs so that he can not only remove the symptoms of illness, but also find its underlying cause. This time factor is another reason for the underuse of this treatment method. The traditional general practitioner, because he is too rushed, coping with too many patients, is often able to spend only five to ten minutes with each individual. Obviously, he would be unable to learn much about a patient in this brief time span, and must, of necessity, be forced to treat the symptom rather than the whole person.

The homoeopathic practitioner who does take the careful case study, prescribes for a patient by using a *Materia Medica* which lists all homoeopathic remedies. He attempts to find the one most similar to the symptoms displayed. Usually a tripod of indications, the three-legged stool, is sought, one of which should be a 'general' characteristic, one a 'mental' characteristic and one a 'specific' characteristic. By a general, I mean a symptom like: 'I am timid', while a 'specific' means a particular feature: 'My arm has a sharp pain.'

Chris Harrington, the three year old we met earlier, provides an illustration of this idea. *Bryonia* was the remedy selected to help 'cure' him. His constipation was regarded as a 'specific' symptom. In addition, Chris was very irritable, a 'mental', and also felt very thirsty, a 'general'. With these indications, *Bryonia* seemed a likely choice. If it had failed, other remedies with at least three indications would have been sought. Some practitioners prefer to use a 'four-legged stool' where at least four definite symptoms are needed before a remedy will be prescribed.

Marjorie Wallace, for instance, was a very fearful person, frightened of the dark, of sudden noises and of being alone. Her illness, a fever, came on very suddenly, accompanied by great thirst, alternate feelings of being hot, then cold, great pain in her head, dizziness, earache and dimness of vision. All these symptoms suggested *Aconitum* which effected a rapid cure.

If you wish to prescribe for yourself, then, you will need to purchase a homoeopathic *Materia Medica*, such as that written by Boericke, against which you can match your own symptoms. It is quite exciting really, this search for remedies which help the body to heal itself. As Stephenson puts it: 'Homoeopathic medicines are ideal for home treatment as they are safe, gentle, pleasant-tasting, cheap, painless, naturally stimulative, and good for most illnesses and for all members of your family (including the pets!).'

The basis of prescribing, then, is seeking to find a remedy listed as being suitable for treatment of at least three or four of your symptoms. However, it is usually a waste of time to use remedies which, while they may superficially match a person's symptoms, do not also match his temperament. Thus, a fair, mild person, given to weepiness would be admirably suited by *Pulsatilla*, an excellent remedy for a wide range of physical symptoms such as acute indigestion, enuresis, hives, and diarrhoea. Conversely a wiry, dark irritable person would be likely to respond to *Nux vomica* whatever the symptoms might be. Similarly, remedies like *Chamomilla*, particularly valuable for teething troubles, swollen abdomen, and coughing, and

Ignatia, excellent for a person who is grieving, would be unlikely to succeed with a person who is calm during illness. They work better with the highly strung individual. So, the section in the *Materia Medica* headed 'Mind' is of particular importance when selecting an appropriate remedy, for most disease or disharmony starts in the mind.

A person's reaction to temperature is also a valuable indicator. Some symptoms are aggravated by the cold, and the person who becomes worse when chilled is likely to be helped by the *Calciums, Arsenicum, Causticum, Phosphorus* and *Rhus tox*. The individual whose symptoms become worse through heat should look to *Argentum nitricum, Natrum muriaticum* (which is common salt), *Pulsatilla* and *Sulphur*. So ask yourself whether you are happier in cold weather or hot. Go further in your self-questioning. Do you fear thunder? Do you prefer to be alone or with others? When ill do you prefer to be alone, or do you like others to fuss over you? Such personal characteristics are of value in finding homoeopathic remedies which will help you as you search the *Materia Medica*.

POTENCY AND DOSAGE

Once a possible remedy is located, the next decision to make involves potency and dosage. Potency relates to the number of dilutions and succussions in the preparation of the remedies. There is considerable disagreement among homoeopaths on the most suitable strength to use. On occasions, they completely contradict one another. For the beginner, the 6X or 12X potency seems a safe one, particularly as it may be repeated at short intervals should it be necessary. For an acute illness, such as influenza, doses of *Gelsemium* (yellow jasmine) may often prove successful in promoting recovery and these could be repeated at half-hourly or hourly intervals.

The guiding rule is to stop administration of a remedy when relief is obtained. Should the improvement cease, then further doses could be taken. With a chronic illness, such as rheumatism, a single dose of high potency, 30X or even 200X, could be given. I would suggest, however, that it is preferable to stay with the low or medium potencies ranging from ∅, which is the mother tincture, to 12X, and use more frequent doses. The more urgent the situation the less time between doses, though for most cases of a non-urgent nature, two or three doses a day seems to be an effective treatment schedule.

THEORIES AND THEORIES

I've mentioned that homoeopaths differ on dosages and potencies. They differ on other points, too, but generally subscribe to the basic theory that sees remedies as single, uncompounded animal, vegetable or mineral substances, which should be administered one at a time. This concept of a single remedy matched to the specific symptom pattern of an individual is, as I have previously pointed out, a stumbling block for general practitioners who lack the time to take the necessary detailed case studies. To overcome this problem, Dr Reckeweg in West Germany has developed a different approach to homoeopathic prescribing which violates the 'single compound theory'. He uses compound remedies in which various homoeopathic substances producing similar compensating effects have been blended together. These compounds are then used like normal drugs to 'cure' a specific illness, not as single remedies to 'cure' a person. Thus a combination of *Aconitum, Bryonia, Eupatorium, Gelsemium, Causticium, Camphora* and *Eucalyptus* are used as an influenza remedy. The theory is that though an individual's symptoms may not match all these substances, one or another will prove effective. It works on the 'shotgun' principle, and has been severely criticized on these grounds by traditional homoeopaths. However, this approach does have the advantage of allowing a practitioner or an individual wanting to treat himself to simply look up the specific remedy for his particular ailment. Unfortunately, as yet, there is no published listing of this nature, but homoeopathic practitioners would be able to supply details to interested enquirers.

As I mentioned earlier, theories explaining why things work have to be tested by yourself rather than taking the word of others. I remember reading about the virtues of chewing honeycomb as a cold preventative measure. Greatly enthused, I began chewing honeycomb only to come down with a dreadful cold a few days later. Similarly with herbal teas which are of undoubted benefit to many people. With me, they produce a cold almost immediately and I prefer to be without colds. Accordingly, I do not use herbal teas. I suggest you use the same approach to homoeopathic remedies, keeping a record of those which help you, and those which seem to have no effect.

You may have noticed that throughout this chapter I have mentioned particular remedies as being useful for specific ailments. This procedure is opposed to homoeopathic theory which maintains a remedy must be matched to a person, not an illness. Yet the Reckeweg approach of using compounds to treat a particular illness seems to work well. Therefore, it would appear useful to identify those remedies which, over many years, have proven successful in helping the body heal certain ailments. This will be of assistance to the person reading this book who does not want to take a careful inventory of his symptoms and search the *Materia Medica* for a possible remedy. Such a person might like to try the remedies suggested. For example, should he develop a sudden cold through getting wet and sitting around in damp clothes, *Dulcamara* is likely to prove helpful. Thus he can try it out for himself, as he has nothing to lose. Should it work, his cold will improve dramatically. If it doesn't, he is no worse off. Accordingly, the next chapter concerns itself with a 'first-aid' approach to homoeopathy, looking at a number of remedies which have proven to be of value in treating quite specific ailments.

To complete the present chapter, I list a number of rules for using homoeopathic medicines which it is wise to observe if their full benefit is to be attained:

1. Store remedies in a cool place away from direct sunlight, perfumes, disinfectants and camphor.
2. Avoid the use of coffee, alcohol, tobacco and spicy foods while treating yourself with homoeopathic remedies. However, you may still take medically prescribed drugs at

the same time without seriously reducing their effect.

3. Take the remedy in a clean mouth, at least 15 minutes before and after eating. Rinsing the mouth with water before taking the medicine is helpful but do not use toothpaste before dosing yourself.

These rules are few, and simple to observe. They will assist you to make the most of your self-help approach. One of the things you will enjoy most is the low cost of your treatment, for the remedies, available from homoeopaths and naturopaths, are cheap and, as they do not spoil, will last for years. In fact, whenever one of my bottles becomes nine-tenths empty, I fill it with rain water, add a few drops of alcohol and succuss it by hitting it against my palm 15 times. Thus, instead of a 6X potency, I now have a 7X potency. It would certainly be difficult to find a self-help medical system as cheap as that.

4. Homoeopathic First Aid

THE 'GREAT REMEDIES'

Judy Tremaine fell down the stairs at her home. Badly bruised and shocked, she reached for a particular homoeopathic remedy. Bob Mason used the same remedy before and after his regular Saturday football match. Lyn Peters took four hourly doses the day before her stomach operation and continued this dosage for three days afterwards. The remedy these people had in common: *Arnica*, one of the great homoeopathic medicines. Where bruising and shock is involved, *Arnica* reigns supreme, just as *Calendula* is excellent for cuts, *Urtica urens* for burns, *Ledum* for stings, *Nux vomica* for stomach upsets, *Sulphur* for skin complaints, *Gelsemium* for influenza, *Arsenicum album* for gastro-enteritis, *Aconite* for sudden chills, and *Bryonia* and *Rhus toxicodendron* for rheumatic pains. All these time proven remedies will be discussed in more detail as this chapter unfolds but, to begin, we'll look at the remedy many homoeopaths consider as the 'greatest'—*Arnica*.

ARNICA

It is particularly valuable in cases of shock, whether this be physical or mental. In emergencies such as heart attacks, car accidents or a severe sporting injury, try to get *Arnica* into the sufferer quickly as a first aid measure while awaiting medical treatment. Surgical operations, be they medical or dental, come under this shock category also. As mentioned in a previous chapter, Margery Blackie places great store in *Arnica* used before and after operations to combat shoch, reduce tissue damage, restore a normal sleep pattern and speed up the healing process. Her book, *The Patient Not the Cure,* recounts cases in which this treatment has proven very successful.

It is particularly interesting that *Arnica* can promote healing retrospectively. Bill Joyce is a case in point. He was involved in a bad car accident and had never really felt well since that time. *Arnica* was instrumental in the improvement of his health so that the negative effects of the past trauma, the accident, were overcome.

Bruising, as long as the skin is unbroken, is another area where *Arnica* is supreme. As well as being taken internally, it can be applied externally as an ointment or as a lotion, with ten drops of the mother tincture (∅) added to half a glass of warm or cold water. The faster the treatment is begun the better the results. On one occasion I had a heavy fall while playing squash. I was unable to save myself and my hip took the full force of the impact. I applied *Arnica* ointment within the hour and again going to bed in the evening. In addition, I took doses of *Arnica* 12X every three hours. On the following day I played a tennis final with no trace of stiffness in the hip, nor was there any sign of bruising.

Virtually all cases of pain and swelling due to bruising, sprained joints, strains, and muscle injuries, can usually be alleviated with *Arnica*. If no beneficial results are noticeable after forty-eight hours of treatment, *Bellis*, a remedy I mentioned in the previous chapter, might be tried as an alternative. This remedy also works well before and after operations. It has particular applicability when a person has been suddenly and unexpectedly immersed in cold water.

There are a number of interesting, quite specific uses for *Arnica* which have been reported by grateful 'patients' over the years. One of these is illustrated by Bob Mason whom I mentioned at the beginning of this chapter. If *Arnica* is taken, say 3–4 times hourly, the day before and the day after a sporting event, the usual stiffness and soreness is either greatly reduced or absent. This is due to the beneficial effect this remedy has on aching and tired limbs. In fact, in any situation where a person is very tired, either through sport, travel, overwork or through spending a sleepless night, *Arnica* is likely to be of help. For those of us who travel frequently over long distances, it is a real blessing, preventing the physical and mental fatigue which is so much a part of this way of life. Actually, *Arnica* can have a vitalizing effect, and it has been used as a 'tonic', taken 2–3 times daily over a period of 2–3 weeks to restore energy. This mode of treatment is particularly valuable after illness, and when elderly people feel weak and dizzy.

Even corns caused by wearing tight shoes can benefit from the application of *Arnica* as long as the skin is unbroken. Where a wound is open, either *Hamamelis* or *Calendula* is a more suitable remedy. Apart from its value in healing cuts, *Hamamelis*, taken both internally and externally, is also an excellent remedy for both varicose veins and haemorrhoids.

CALENDULA

Just as *Arnica* reigns supreme with bruising, *Calendula* is the sovereign remedy for broken skin, particularly when it is necessary to stop bleeding. *Calendula* ointment soothes and promotes rapid healing of cuts, skin cracks, chapped hands, and small septic spots. A lotion of ten drops of *Calendula* mother tincture to half a cup of warm water is an excellent antiseptic and provides a very satisfactory dressing for wounds. Bleeding may be staunched by drops of the mother tincture applied to the affected areas, and healing is accelerated if the remedy is also taken internally. Although *Calendula* is generally effective with nose bleeds, another remedy, *Vipera*, to be repeated every fifteen minutes, might work faster.

Where the eye is troubled by dust or a foreign body, two drops of *Calendula* to forty ml of water provides an excellent eyewash, as does *Euphrasia*, used externally and internally. Similarly, burns in the mouth, a result of taking in food or drink which is too hot, may be soothed by a mixture of ten drops of *Calendula* to half a glass of water. This preparation is sipped and held in the mouth every few minutes. A blend of *Calendula* and

Urtica urens in ointment form is an effective treatment for most small burns, being applied after the injured part has been placed under the cold water tap. This ointment can be very soothing for sunburn and various types of eczemas, often promoting quite rapid healings.

URTICA URENS

This remedy, prepared from the stinging nettle, is perhaps the most widely effective of the homoeopathic burn remedies. It is taken both internally and externally. Twenty drops to a large cup of water provides a lotion in which a pad of gauze might be soaked. This is applied to the burn, covered with lint and cotton wool, then bandaged. It normally relieves the pain of burns very quickly and is a suitable first aid treatment. However, with serious burns, do not apply ointments or lotions until medical advice is available.

While talking of burns remedies, I should mention *Causticum* which is particularly valuable when healing is very slow. Some burns show no signs of healing and it is in such cases that *Causticum* might provide the solution. It has other applications also, being of use when a person becomes very hoarse or actually loses his voice. Singers, lecturers, preachers or anyone who uses his or her voice a great deal would benefit from having this remedy available in the family medicine chest. *Causticum* can also play an important part in preventing the retention of urine after an operation and has proven to be of value in the treatment of cystitis.

As would be expected from its name, stinging nettle, *Urtica urens* is particularly efficacious as a healing agent in cases of nettlerash. In fact, whenever a person has been stung by any sort of plant, this remedy is likely to bring relief. Bee stings, too, yield to *Urtica urens*, though *Ledum*, the next remedy to be discussed, is generally considered to be the first choice in this situation. However, *Urtica urens* could be thought of in cases of hives and gout. The action of the remedy is to reduce the uric acid level in the blood, thus helping the body to rid itself of these troublesome ailments which are often rather resistant to conventional medical treatment.

LEDUM

It is not only bee stings which *Ledum* treats so effectively. The discomfort of most animal and insect bites is quickly relieved by internal and external applications, as is the pain of puncture wounds from sharp pointed instruments such as nails. If *Ledum* is taken as soon as possible after the injury, sepsis is prevented. Some homoeopaths would go so far as to claim that rapid treatment with this remedy prevents tetanus, but I think it more advisable to seek medical assistance in the form of an antitetanus injection. However, as a first-aid measure, obviously *Ledum* would be very helpful. With painful puncture wounds and injuries such as a splinter under the nail, *Ledum* may be taken internally whenever the pain returns. It can be taken at half-hourly intervals should it prove necessary. Further relief from pain may be achieved by a lotion of ten drops of *Ledum* to half a cup of cold water applied as a dressing to the wound. Another use of such a dressing would be in the case of a 'black eye' where quick relief is usually obtainable.

Quite a different attribute of this remedy is its function as an antidote to the effect of whisky. However, *Coffea*, which is made from coffee, is probably a better all purpose remedy if 'sobering-up' is necessary. It is also useful for insomnia, where the cause of sleeplessness is over-excitability.

NUX VOMICA

Nux vomica mentioned in the previous chapter, is also a 'hangover' remedy for the nervous, irritable, dark person who has overindulged. Indigestion, wind in the stomach, gastric upsets due to overeating, and colic are all relieved by this remedy, though vomiting and nausea are better treated with *Ipecacuanha*. A very good indication as to whether a person will benefit from the use of *Nux vomica* is his sensitivity level, for it is a useful treatment for those of us who 'cannot stand' sensations such as loud noise, strong smells and bright lights.

Usually people who do react badly to such stimuli tend to be rather nervous and anxious, so *Nux vomica* is often valuable in relieving nervous headache and neuritis. It is one of the most valuable 'nerve' remedies along with *Kali phos.* and *Argentum nitricum.* These three homoeopathic medicines have proven themselves over the years as 'relaxants', helping people cope more serenely with their lives. Yet they produce none of the undesirable side effects and dependence of our modern tranquillizers such as Librium and Valium. It is worth pointing out, too, that *Nux vomica* is an effective de-toxicant, clearing the system after drugs or anaesthetics have been taken.

Actually this remedy, and most of the others discussed in this chapter, are referred to as polycrests. A polycrest has a healing effect on a wide range of ailments, so it is not surprising that I suggest *Nux vomica* for so many health problems. Even insomnia comes within its scope, particularly when the sleeplessness is a result of drinking coffee.

Another member of the *Nux* family, *Nux moschata*, which is a remedy derived from nutmeg, has the opposite effect, for it can be used to combat sleepiness. For those of us who tend to fall asleep during talks or while reading, this can be a valuable means of remedying our drowsy state. It can be of help, too, in alleviating the weakness of old age. *Phosphoric acid* can be used in the same way together with *Conium maculatum* which is particularly indicated for memory weakness. Where the weakness is in children rather than older people, *Baryta carbynica* might be tried instead.

SULPHUR

This remedy can be of value in children's complaints when it is the skin which is causing concern. Various types of infantile eczema have yielded to its healing power though skin problems are notoriously difficult to treat. Our drug-oriented medical treatment has been singularly unsuccessful in this area so nothing is really being lost if *Sulphur* is tried first.

Actually, this remedy has often been considered as one of the most important in the homoeopath's kit. Stephenson, whose book was referred to earlier, quotes an old teacher of his who told him, only half in jest, that he could practice homoeopathy with three remedies—*Sepia* for the ladies, *Sulphur* for the men, and *Arnica* for injuries. There is no doubt that these three remedies do have extremely wide effects, and might often be used as a first approach to treatment. In my own experience, I have not made great use of *Sulphur* but we all have our favourite remedies—many practitioners swear by its healing power. Certainly in the area of skin troubles it is considered to be the remedy most likely to succeed, though its range of application extends from bowel and stomach disturbances through haemorrhoids to summer heat complaints.

There are other homoeopathic remedies, of course, which might be used if *Sulphur* is unable to improve troublesome skin conditions. *Petroleum* and *Graphites*, for example, are alternative treatments for infantile eczema. The latter can also be helpful in cases of gastric pains, wind and distension. Ringworm frequently yields to *Tellurium*, chilblains to *Agaricus*, and septic pimples to *Arnica*. Should pus and matter be present, *Hepar sulph*. is likely to produce improvement.

All the above remedies are useful in other areas too, *Tellurium*, for instance, often being used to counter offensive footsweat, and *Petroleum* serving as a remedy for travel sickness. Alternative travel sickness remedies are *Cocculus* and *Tabacum*, the latter being prepared from tobacco. These should be taken one dose nightly for three to four days before travelling and a dose at the first sign of discomfort during the journey.

GELSEMIUM

Gelsemium is known as an excellent remedy for influenza, its distinguishing feature being that the sufferer is not thirsty. If he is thirsty, *Bryonia* or *Eupatorum* would be better remedies to try first. This choice of medicine in terms of a patient's own reaction relates back to a point stressed earlier, homoeopathy treats people, not just illnesses. All of us become sick differently. One person with flu gets hot, another is chilly, while a third has aches all over her body. For each of these people, a different remedy is likely to be most effective. It is very satisfying to diagnose yourself in order to find the particular 'medicine picture' which fits your particular symptoms but, if you do not wish to do so, I would suggest *Gelsemium* as the first remedy to try if you have influenza.

It is also a helpful remedy if you are suffering from heat exhaustion. *Sulphur*, of course, helps, too, in this situation. Should you develop a throbbing headache as a result of sunstroke, *Glonoine* can provide relief. It is an excellent treatment for anyone likely to be upset by sun and heat. All the above remedies help with weakness brought on by hot weather. So, too, does *Selenium* which may be used whenever you overexert yourself physically or mentally.

Another use for *Gelsemium* includes its function as a 'nerve' remedy, and it has often been employed to calm students with examination fear. However, I prefer *Argentum nitricum* in this situation as it seems to remove fears of many kinds. People frightened of public speaking, or of meeting strangers, or of going out shopping alone are all helped by this remedy. As mentioned earlier, *Kali phos.*, is also extremely good in this area, being one of the really great nerve remedies.

Many people swear by *Gelsemium* as a cold preventative. A student of mine, Tom Ballant, would always take this remedy for three or four nights after he had been in touch with anyone who had a cold.

ARSENICUM ALBUM

This medicine is also widely used as a cold preventative, taken in the same way as Tom took his *Gelsemium*. It has been found valuable in the treatment of hay fever where there is incessant sneezing. *Alium cepa*, the common onion, is an alternative remedy likely to be useful with this complaint. Though *Arsenicum album* has claimed considerable success with asthma sufferers, *Arum triphyllum* might be a more effective remedy for this particular ailment. Should sinusitis be the problem rather than hay fever or asthma, *Silica* could provide relief.

One of the key indicators that a person might benefit from *Arsenicum album* is fearfulness. Lynda Bales is such a person. She fears almost everything, spending her waking hours in worry and anxiety, apprehensively awaiting the next blow. Naturally enough, she possesses a wide spectrum of physical symptoms too, including burning pains in the stomach, constant gastric upsets, headaches and diarrhoea. Mentally she is irritable and depressed. Or rather, she was. Several doses of *Arsenicum album* 6X greatly reduced the fearfulness and, over a period of several months, the other symptoms gradually disappeared. Lynda's case supports the homoeopathic theory that the minute dose stimulates the body to heal itself so that once improvement begins, the remedy can be discontinued to let nature take its course. This remedy is *the* choice for gastroenteritis, food poisoning, vomiting and diarrhoea, and is a particularly valuable one to take with you when you travel.

Where children become overexcited in anticipation of some future event, a single dose of *Arsenicum album* can be very effective in exerting a calming influence. Perhaps, this same influence is part of the reason why it is so often effective in another area involving 'nerves', namely shingles.

ACONITE

It should, by now, have become obvious that there exists a considerable overlap between the various remedies. Different remedies can serve as treatments for the same ailment, and a single remedy can ameliorate many ailments at the same time. So there is really no substitute for self-experimentation, finding out what works for you.

Aconite, like *Arsenicum*, helps frightened people. This fear can take the form of a general agitation, a sense of unease, or a more specific fear such as might be reflected in children's nightmares. The person who experiences such a state is usually oversensitive, starts easily, and maintains a high degree of tension, both physical and mental. *Aconite* can help such a person become less frightened and in so doing clear up a spectrum of physical symptoms like coughs, colds, inflamed eyes, swollen legs, and kidney problems.

However, this remedy's main sphere of action lies in sudden chills. It is of great value in the early stages of a fever or chill which has come on very quickly, perhaps during exposure to 'dry cold' and winds. 'Wet cold' would find *Dulcamara* a more appropriate remedy. Frequently a person will return from watching, say, a football match, chilled to the bone and trembling with cold. Several doses of *Aconite* given at half-hourly or hourly intervals would probably prevent the chill developing. That is, *Aconite's* influence is great at the beginning of illness. Once the illness becomes established it is necessary to seek other remedies. For example, should you start feeling the first effects of a summer stomach upset, that is the time to use *Aconite*. It is no use waiting until you have a fully fledged stomach ache. Similarly with toothaches caused by cold or a draught, check them early, and you may find they never develop into a serious problem.

BRYONIA

This remedy has been mentioned already, both in terms of its effectiveness in 'curing' constipation and its value as an influenza remedy when the patient is very thirsty and aches all over. It can be alternated with *Eupatorium* to cope with this type of influenza.

However, Bryonia's main use as a 'specific' is for the relief of rheumatic pains. Backaches, stiff joints, swollen limbs and painful shoulders all benefit greatly from *Bryonia,* as do coughs where the pain is deep in the chest. The main indicator for its use is that the patient feels better for rest. If your elbow aches badly as you use your arm, but feels more comfortable when you are in bed, then *Bryonia* is for you. However, if your legs ache while you are in bed but become more comfortable as you get up and move about, this remedy is unlikely to help you.

RHUS TOXICODENDRON

Rhus tox. complements *Bryonia* by helping when the rheumatic pains become better through movement. Where the stiffness in joints and tendons, the lumbago, the fibrositis all become easier and more comfortable as you walk about and use your body, *Rhus tox.* is the remedy most likely to be of assistance. You will feel this to be particularly true when your stiffness and soreness is due to exposure to dampness. Similarly if you catch a cold through becoming wet, *Rhus tox.* is likely to aid your recovery. *Dulcarama* as mentioned earlier, also provides relief under those conditions.

Sporting injuries such as strained muscles, ligaments and tendons which feel better as you warm them through movement will respond to *Rhus tox*. An external treatment for sprains, ten drops of the remedy to half a glass of warm water, applied as a lotion can be very helpful, particularly if combined with internal treatment of dosage at 3–4 hourly intervals.

SOME OTHER USEFUL REMEDIES

In addition to the key remedies so far described, there are many others which are of great value in coping with specific ailments. Most people, though not all, will find these effective.

One of my favourites is *Pulsatilla* which helps in cases of indigestion from rich food, headaches due to overwork, postnatal depression, delayed menstruation, measles, and rheumatism which occurs in a single joint such a knee or elbow. An excellent indication for the use of this remedy is the desire for loose clothing. Tight belts, in particular, are found to be intolerable. *Pulsatilla* is particularly suited for pale, quiet people who are shy and retiring, maybe rather weepy on occasions. Homoeopaths, oblivious of the charge of sexism which might be levelled against them, refer to it primarily as a female remedy.

They view *Sepia* in the same way, for this remedy is widely considered as perhaps the greatest homoeopathic remedy for female complaints. Often it works best for thin, dark women and is particularly helpful in menstruation problems and anaemia. *Caulophyllum,* too, can be of use in relieving menstrual pain. It has often been employed by expectant mothers for a month before delivery to ease the discomfort of childbirth. Sexual problems, where a woman complains of the pain of intercourse or of loss of interest in intercourse, can often be resolved quickly through the use of *Sepia*. More broadly, this remedy can help where a person becomes hostile towards loved ones for no apparent reason.

Where men have sexual problems, such as loss of sexual desire, poor erections and impotency, *Lycopedium* is an excellent homoeopathic remedy to try. It has also proven of value in cases of falling hair and insomnia. Where a person is unduly tired, finding work a burden, *Lycopedium* is likely to improve matters. This is particularly so if the person is depressed and down in health at the same time. However, for depression I have found *Aurum metallicum* to be the remedy which consistently helps most people. That would be my first choice, with *Lycopedium* my second and *Lilium tigrinum*, the tiger lily, my third. All three remedies have proven successful in alleviating hopelessness, despair, suicidal tendencies and general mental misery. It is, once again, a matter of finding the one which brings you, personally, the improvement you seek.

Lycopedium is a right-sided remedy. That is, it tends to be most effective in cases where ailments develop first on the right hand side of the body. Sore throats which begin on the right side, for example, and joint pains which tend to localize in the right ankle, knee, elbow or shoulder. *Lachesis*, on the other hand, is a left-sided remedy which is particularly valuable where sore throats and pain begin on this side of the body. This remedy is *the* treatment for menopausal problems such as hot flushes, weeping, heart palpitations and faintness. It works best for women who are worse for warmth, *Sepia* perhaps being a better choice for those who are worse for cold. However, one or the other of these two remedies should bring relief from the discomforts of the menopause. *Lachesis* has other applications also, chief among them being the treatment of shingles, acute thrombosis and post-partum complaints. The person who cannot bear tight clothing and whose complaints are worse after sleep is likely to benefit greatly from this remedy.

Jill Rogers did not feel worse after sleep, but her migraine certainly did become more intense whenever she visited the seaside. This is a strong indication that *Natrum muriaticum*, or common salt, would be helpful to Jill in 'curing' her migraine. This remedy is useful in treating colds, where there is violent sneezing; coughs, where there is a pain in the head as a result of the coughing; and bed-wetting. It is an excellent remedy for shock and can lead to mood improvement in people who are resentful that life has not treated them better.

The effectiveness of *Natrum muriaticum* in modifying the negative emotional state of resentment is typical of the way in which homoeopathic medicine helps the mind as well as the body. Another example of this is *Ignatia* which usually assists people to cope more easily with grief. Where a person becomes hysterical through grief or shock, *Ignatia* can bring sudden improvement. *Phosphoric acid* is another remedy which produces similar benefits.

Hypericum is also a medicine of value in combating the effects of shock or fright. Its main use, however, lies in its relief of intense pain. Where nerves are injured, as when a finger is crushed in a door, *Hypericum* is the remedy of choice. It is good for any type of crush injury to finger or toe, in which situation, a solution of ten drops to half a cup of warm water may be used to soak the affected part; for any wound, no matter how small, which is acutely painful; for operations and dental extractions; for spinal injuries involving nerve damage; for pain in the coccyx; for alleviating the pain of amputated limbs; and for shingles. Septic wounds, grazes and abrasions, stings and punctures where pain shoots up the nerves of the limb from the damaged area, are all helped by the remedy. The key indications are acute pain and injury to nerves.

Great pain is also a characteristic of symptoms calling for *Belladona*. Throbbing headaches, toothache, earache when the ear is red and hot, heavy, painful periods with low back pain, bright red flow and a feeling that the insides are being dragged out, boils with a hot throbbing red area around the boil, and lymphangitis with the characteristic red streaks up the arm, all yield to *Belladonna*'s healing effect. The key symptom is redness, usually combined with heat and throbbing pain.

Bone pain is a main indicator for the use of *Ruta*. Where bones are bruised or broken this remedy is the first choice. Combined in an accident mixture with equal parts of *Arnica* and *Symphytom*, it may be used to cover virtually everything from a simple fall to a fracture. Even eyeball injuries can be helped with this accident remedy. *Ruta* used alone has wide applicability, having been successfully employed externally as an ointment for sprained or strained joints and ligaments; for rheumatic conditions where a person feels sore and bruised; for eyestrain due to much reading and studying; for pain in enlarged joints; for 'housemaid's knee' and 'tennis elbow'; for broken chilblains; and for piles. Its primary action is upon wrenched and torn tendons, split ligaments and joints. Youngsters who develop strains through too active play or who receive a kick on the shin during a football match have reason to bless *Ruta*'s healing power.

Similarly, the person who suffers from gastric pains, wind and stomach distension blesses *Carbo vegetabilis*. The swollen abdomen tends to subside under its influence and the belching either disappears or, at least, is greatly reduced. *Carbo veg.* is valuable in cases of food poisoning, particularly when bad fish is the culprit, or when a person feels very ill through eating fatty foods. It also is most effective in aiding recovery after a person has experienced an exhausting illness, and in correcting anaemic conditions. Given as a single 6X or 12X dose every two or three days, *Carbo veg.* has proven its worth as a cold preventative, helping those people with a tendency to have many colds, or those who are still weak after illness.

Should the weakness or illness date back to the time when the person had a vaccination, *Thuja* is the homoeopathic remedy of choice. Many people claim to have never felt really well since a particular vaccination and, for them, *Thuja* will frequently effect a marked improvement in their state of health. It has also been widely used for many years as a curative for warts. Less frequently, it has been employed to assist the bed-wetting child in overcoming his uncomfortable habit.

Chamomilla has been used in this way, also, but its main claim to fame in the homoeopathic repertoire lies in the relief it brings to teething children. In addition, it is an excellent general remedy, being particularly suitable to children and adults who 'cannot stand' things. Such people complain loudly when in pain, are irritable, tense, and impatient. *Chamomilla* is not a remedy, therefore, to use with the quiet, stoical individual.

Two final 'specifics' are *Berberis*, which has a long record of success in dissolving kidney stones, and *Phytolacca* which reigns supreme as a sore throat remedy. For hoarseness or loss of voice, take *Phytolacca* internally and gargle with a mixture of ten drops to half a glass of water.

GENERAL INDICATORS

On first reading, you may experience some confusion over which remedy is best for you. All those described in this chapter have been successful for many years in promoting healing without producing harmful side effects. If you stick to the 6X or 12X potency, you can safely experiment until you find *your* remedies. However, there are some general pointers which might guide your initial choices:

- The *Arsenic type* is careful and tidy about his person and his home, therefore he tends to be immaculately dressed, behaving fastidiously.
- The *Sulphur type* has been dubbed the 'ragged philosopher', for he is untidy in dress and personal habits, often appearing unwashed and unkempt.
- The *Lycopedium type* is the worried executive, grey-haired and often with a deeply lined face.
- The *Pulsatilla type* tends to be a weepy blonde.
- The *Natrum muriaticum type* is the joyful female.
- The *Arnica type* wants to be left alone, does not like being touched, and tends to be indifferent to life's events.
- The *Calcarea carbonica type* is fat, flabby and very pale.
- The *Belladonna type* has glowing red cheeks and a dry, burning skin.
- The *Chamomilla type* just 'can't beat it', whatever 'it' may be.

According to Margery Blackie, to whom I have earlier referred, a person's handshake may reveal the key to his or her constitutional remedy. This constitutional medicine is the one most suitable for treating a particular individual in the sum total of his mental, emotional and physical strengths and weaknesses. Once you identify your own remedy you will find it improves your health virtually irrespective of your particular symptoms. So perhaps you can inquire of people who know you what your handshake is like.

- A cold dry hand indicates *Arsenicum*.
- A cold damp hand suggests *Hepar sulph*.
- A rough, cracked hand indicates *Silica*.
- A cold, damp, limp hand suggests *Calcarea carbonica*.
- A firm handshake indicates *Lycopedium*.
- A profusely sweating hand suggests *Thuja*.

These last two chapters have provided an overview of a well-tried system of self-help medicine. Enough information is given to enable you to get started on an adventure in self-healing which may pay enormous dividends in the improvement of your health without recourse to drugs. Hopefully, you will want to go further, to find out more about homoeopathy, perhaps through reading or talking with a homoeopathic practitioner or naturopath, but, whether you do or not, you should enjoy healing yourself with the 'hair of the dog'. Just as the whisky drinker combats his hangover by drinking whisky next day, and the doctor uses an injection of a weakened strain of influenza virus to vaccinate against influenza, you can use minute quantities of a substance to cure illnesses which would be caused by large doses of the same substance. Like cures like, and I hope you find it cures you.

5. Bach Flower Remedies

BACH'S THEORY OF DISEASE

Another system of self-help medicine, available from homoeopaths and naturopaths which is easy to administer, is that developed by Dr Edward Bach during the 1930s. Abandoning a profitable Harley Street practice due to his disenchantment with the orthodox medicine of the time, Bach sought a system of medicine which would heal the sick without generating any adverse side-effects. His observations, both in his career as a house surgeon and as a bacteriologist, led to the conclusion that no two people with the same disease reacted in the same way. One might be impatient, another passive and long-suffering, while a third might be frightened. A similar variety of reactions was observable in ostensibly well people. Thus, Bach decided that it was a person's mental state which was all-important rather than the physical symptoms he might display.

He theorized that the basis of disease lay in the disharmony of conflicting moods which produced unhappiness, mental torture, lethargy, fear and resignation. Such disharmony lowered the body's vitality, permitting disease to flourish. Accordingly, Bach sought remedies which would act on and modify the mood and temperament of the patient rather than remedies which would treat the physical symptoms. He shared the homoeopathic view that as each person is different, he must be treated for his personal mood and the need of the moment, irrespective of any particular disease from which he might be suffering.

So Bach's simple and effective system of healing is based on the premise that it is our anxieties, our fears and our cares which open up our bodies to the invasion of disease, a theory quite similar to that of modern experts like Hans Selye who see stress as the basic element in making us vulnerable to illness. By treating our fears and anxieties, Bach argued that not only would we free ourselves from our physical symptoms, but we would also feel happier in ourselves.

John Hardie would certainly agree. Only a young man, he was plagued by splitting headaches. He was also tortured by jealousy. Whenever his girlfriend was out of his sight, he was prey to dark forebodings, suspicions crowding his mind until he was unable to concentrate on his work or on anything else. His whole life was disrupted by his headaches and his jealousy which he seemed quite unable to control. *Holly*, one of the Bach remedies, was prescribed, three drops in a little water four times a day. According to John, within three days the jealousy began easing and by the end of the first week he was functioning quite normally. He felt much more settled within himself and the headaches of which he had complained seemed to have vanished. However, he did continue the holly treatment for three weeks to be on the safe side.

Bach believed that in illness a change of mood occurs in the patient. He is different from the way he ordinarily is, and this difference of mood provides a guide to the necessary remedy or remedies. Because the mind is the most sensitive part of the body, it shows the onset and the course of the disease much more definitely than does the body. Chancellor, in his *Handbook of the Bach Flower Remedies*, stresses the preventive value of this approach, pointing out that just as moods provide a guide to the treatment of illness, they also warn us that a complaint is imminent and enable us to stop the attack before it develops. That is, a person's mood may change before, and sometimes long before, the disease appears, enabling us to take preventive measures.

Beth Sanders, normally an energetic, cheerful woman, started coming home from her teaching job in a resentful, embittered mood. Her usual sunny disposition was noticeable by its absence and she was just 'not herself'. To one versed in the Bach approach this 'unlike self' condition provides an advance warning of physical illness on the way. Three drops of *Willow* taken in a little water three times a day restored Beth's cheerfulness within a week and no physical illness developed.

We may claim that the Bach remedy had aborted the disease before it could develop. This is one possibility. However, a critic of the Bach system could claim, equally justifiably, that Beth was simply out of sorts, and that her mood change had nothing to do with any impending illness. The fact that no disease developed 'proves' that she was not sickening for something.

We cannot know which of these views is correct in Beth's case. No illness appeared, but was this because of the remedy or because there was no illness? However, in many cases documented by Chancellor, illnesses did develop if changed mood states were not treated. We can be our own experts on this. Observe yourself and note those times when 'you are not yourself'. See what happens. Do symptoms of physical illness appear? If so, you have nothing to lose by using the appropriate Bach remedies in future cases. They are harmless, having no side effects, and may possibly be very helpful.

In fact, the situation is similar to that when we take Vitamin C as a cold preventative. At the first signs of cold, many people take one gram of Vitamin C and repeat the dose hourly for a day. Usually, no cold develops and the symptoms disappear. The critic can say there is no evidence that the cold would ever have appeared. However, all he has to do is investigate for himself, by sometimes taking Vitamin C and by sometimes doing nothing. He will soon find whether this remedy works for him. Adopt the same approach for the Bach remedies. Try them out to find whether you, as an individual, can 'head off' illness by being guided by your unusual mood changes.

Of course, all of us experience passing mood changes during the day. These influence us to a lesser extent. The common feeling of 'getting out of the wrong side of bed', for example, usually presages a bad day. We tend to be grumpy at breakfast, irritable during the day, and tired at night. Yet a dose of *Impatiens* taken immediately you are aware of your early morning irritability is likely to effect a mood change so your day becomes far more enjoyable. By treating the unhappy state of mind when it occurs, ill humor can often be prevented, and ill health avoided. As Bach put it in *The Twelve Healers:* 'Take no notice of the disease, think only of the outlook on life of the one in distress . . . Disease is but the consolidation of a mental attitude.'

Still, the choice is yours. You may not wish to be particularly good humoured. Some of us enjoy being out of sorts. However, if you do want to modify your more negative mood states, Dr Bach may have provided the answer for you.

PREPARATION OF THE REMEDIES

As with homoeopathy, the great virtue of the Bach flower method is its safety as a self-help medical system. It uses 'essence of flower' as the active agent, with the flowers of specific herbs, shrub and trees being potentized through the use of sunshine. The blooms of the plants Bach identified as 'healers' are picked and immediately floated on the surface of pure water contained in a thin, glass bowl. When the blooms cover the entire surface of the water, they are left in bright sunshine for three or four hours, or until the blooms start to fade. They are then removed from the water which is poured into bottles so as to half fill them. A preservative, brandy, is used to complete the filling of the bottles which then become stock. From these bottles, the homoeopathic pharmacist or health store proprietor takes three drops and makes up the mixture for use by adding distilled water and alcohol. It is this latter preparation that you use to treat yourself. As with homoeopathic remedies, the dose is infinitesimal, yet it would seem to exert healing effects out of all proportion to its volume.

Most of the thirty-eight Bach remedies are prepared by the 'sunshine method' outlined above. Some, however, are the result of the 'boiling method' by which the blossoms, together with small pieces of stem or stalk, and the young, fresh leaves, are boiled for half an hour in clean, pure water. The water is then bottled as with the other method. Whichever of the two methods is used, it is obvious that the whole process is a natural one, uncontaminated by chemical substances. Therefore, even if a Bach remedy is misprescribed, and does not produce healing, no harm results.

DOSAGE

Normally the remedies are taken in their pure and simple form. A person who is, for example, lacking in self-confidence would take *Larch*. However, such a person is likely to be indecisive, and if this is the case, *Scheranthus* and possibly *Cerato*, could be mixed with the *Larch*. If, in addition, this person was also tired, lacking the energy to do his normal tasks, a strengthener such as *Hornbeam* could complete the preparation.

The only ready mixed remedy suggested by Bach was his 'rescue remedy'. It comprises *Star of Bethlehem* for shock, *Rock Rose* for terror and panic, *Impatiens* for mental strain and tension, *Cherry Plum* for desperation, and *Clematis* for the disoriented, vague, out-of-the-body feeling which often precedes loss of consciousness. This remedy may be used fruitfully in any emergency where a person is shocked, frightened, or suffering pain. Three drops are added to a glass of water, the patient sipping this every few minutes. As he improves, his sips become less frequent, say every quarter-hour and then every half-hour. Should the patient be unconscious, and thus unable to sip the water, rub it on his gums, his wrists and behind his ears. If no water is available, use the 'rescue remedy' undiluted to moisten lips, gums and tongue. Once the initial emergency has passed, this remedy may be used over the recovery period with three drops to a teaspoon of water being taken four times a day. It may be used externally to treat wounds. Make a lotion of six drops to half a litre of water and apply it as a hot or cold fomentation.

However, dosage, as with homoeopathic remedies, is really not critical. I've mentioned three drops earlier in this chapter but many people use four, five or even ten drops in a little water, taken three or four times a day. This dosage is suitable for babies, children and adults alike. In cases of acute illness, the dosage may be increased to every quarter-hour, or even more frequently if so desired. The 'medicine' is continued until the patient shows definite improvement, at which time dosage becomes less frequent. Although overdosing does not increase the effectiveness of a remedy, many practitioners who use the Bach system recommend giving four doses a day until well after the patient has recovered. Others follow homoeopathic principles and suggest a cessation once improvement is marked. You will need to experiment for yourself.

It will also be helpful to change remedies during severe illness, for the moods of the patient will change according to the stage his recovery has reached. Perhaps different remedies could be used singly at different times, or you may prefer to combine three, four or five to cover varying mood states.

This type of treatment does not conflict with other methods. Bach stressed that his remedies could be used in conjunction with any other form of treatment without risk of interference, or could be used alone to achieve effective healing. He also stressed that such healing was not to be limited only to humans, for animals and plants responded very positively to the remedies. Many dogs struck by cars and left to suffer on the road have been helped to recovery through the 'rescue remedy', as have plants damaged by storms and rough treatment.

In fact, as with homoeopathy, this positive response on the part of plants has provided something of a stumbling block to critics who claim no active role for the remedies, maintaining any results gained are because the patient 'talks himself into' getting better. Often it is infants, animals, and plants who seem to respond best to the treatment. Further, it does not seem to matter whether the person giving the remedy or the patient taking it has the slightest faith in it.

USE OF THE REMEDIES

Selecting Bach remedies for yourself is easier than prescribing the appropriate homoeopathic remedy which embraces 'generals', 'mind' and 'specifics'. Physical symptoms are ignored, the mood state being the indicator. Some of the more widely used remedies and the mood state which they treat are outlined in the following examples.

Tiredness and irritability are common visitors to modern man. Brendon Mitchell is no exception. He is grumpy before breakfast, is typically cross at work during the day, and unwinds at night by 'blasting' his family. From comments made earlier in this chapter, you'll realize immediately that Brendon should head for the *Impatiens* bottle. However, in addition to his irritability, Brendon is subject to fits of depression. When he feels like this, he can see no light or happiness in his world. *Gentian* would probably help him, and it could be mixed with the *Impatiens*. Should it not lead to an improvement of his mood, *Gentian* might well be replaced by *Mustard*.

Unlike Brendon, Marjorie Patterson presents an outward face of cheerfulness and brightness. She laughs a lot, hums to herself and certainly shows no evidence of her inner state, which is one of real mental torture. Constantly beset by worries over her health and that of her family, tortured by guilt over past mistakes, racked by fears for the future, Marjorie lives a truly miserable life despite the brave face which others see. *Agrimony* is her remedy, one which could relieve the inner misery.

Nancy Callard is not one to conceal her suffering behind a cheerful exterior. Instead she plunges headlong into self-pity, absolutely wallowing in the unhappiness of her life and the injustice of the treatment she receives. *Chicory* is likely to help Nancy emerge from the sea of self-pity and, if she combines it with *Willow*, she may be able to let go of the feeling that life has treated her badly.

Fears beset us all at some time or another and in many cases cause us to live very unhappily. Joan Battersby is frightened of the dark, of being alone, and of growing old. Because she knows of what she is frightened, Joan could find relief in *Mimulus*. However, should she experience vague fears which she cannot pin down, or free-floating anxiety attacks, *Aspen* is more likely to alleviate her condition. When fear becomes real terror though, *Rock Rose* is the remedy to turn to.

Roger Liverman is indecisive, constantly vacillating between two alternatives. First he feels he should do this, then he feels he should do that. Unable to make a decision, he suffers considerable self-imposed mental torment which shows itself in skin problems, rashes, boils and pimples. *Scleranthus* is likely to help him make up his mind, and *Crab Apple*, a cleansing remedy, will possibly alleviate the skin trouble. Should Roger, once he has made his decision, fear that he has made a mistake and so commence worrying anew, *Mimulus* may help him forget his fear. If he is prone to asking the opinion of all and sundry because he doubts his own ability to make a decision, Roger could try *Cerato*.

These cases illustrate the basic principle involved in prescribing Bach remedies for yourself. Observe yourself, and note how you react to certain circumstances. How do you react when you are very tired? Or when confronted by a serious emergency? Or when you have to make an important decision? At such times, the real you emerges from behind your defenses, allowing your true feelings to surface. Stripped of the usual mask of self-justification and excuses, your difficulties can be identified and, once recognized, treated according to the Bach system. As stressed earlier, do not wait for illness to appear but use the appropriate remedies to help you overcome negative states of mind.

DESCRIPTION OF THE REMEDIES

Chancellor, to whom I have referred earlier in this chapter, provides key words such as weak-willed, distrust, desperate, and terror, which sum up the mental states for which a particular remedy is appropriate. Bach, in his booklet *The Twelve Healers and Other Remedies,* gives a short description of the type of person who may be helped by each of the remedies. I have attempted to outline this information in the pages which follow so that a person wishing to use the Bach system can match his or her mood states to the main features of each remedy. These are listed alphabetically:

Agrimony For *mental torture which is concealed from others* behind a mask of cheerfulness and humour. Alcohol or drugs are often used to help bear the suffering. This person loves peace and is distressed by argument.

Aspen For *vague fears of unknown origin, anxiety and apprehension*. Often this person is unable to share fears with others.

Beech For *intolerance, criticism of others*. This person frequently passes harsh judgement upon people, yet feels the need to see more good and beauty in all that surrounds him, and to be more tolerant of the views of others.

Centaury For a kind, gentle person, rather *weak-willed* who is *over-anxious to serve others*. This person is *too easily influenced*, becoming more a servant than a willing helper, giving up personal needs to meet those of others.

Cerato For one who *distrusts himself* and *doubts his own ability*, constantly seeks advice from others, and is often misguided. This person does not have sufficient self-confidence to make his own decisions.

Cherry Plum For one who *fears doing some terrible thing, of losing control of his mind*, who becomes *desperate* because of his dread that his reason will give way.

Chestnut Bud For one who seems to repeat the same mistakes in his life because of his *failure to learn by experience*. This person seems unable to learn the lessons of daily life without considerable repetition.

Chicory For the person who is continually putting things right and *wants his own way*. Such a person tends to be *possessive* and *egotistical* and full of self-love.

Clematis For the *dreamer: indifferent, inattentive, sleepy* and *withdrawn from reality*. A quiet person, not really happy in present circumstances, who lives in hopes of future happier times, and who often makes little effort to recover when sick.

Crab Apple A *cleansing remedy* for the person who feels there is something about their physical or mental state which is not quite clean. This person feels self-disgust, wanting to be free from the one thing (frequently quite trivial) which makes him feel unclean.

Elm For one who is constantly *overstriving for perfection* with an *extreme sense of responsibility*. At times he feels *despondent* because the important task in which he is engaged seems too difficult.

Gentian For one who is *easily discouraged*. Any interference or hindrance to daily activities causes *doubt* and *depression*, and soon disheartens this person.

Gorse For *hopelessness* and *despair*. This person has given up hope that anything can be done to relieve his suffering.

Heather For the *self-centred person* who is so *full of his own concerns* that he must have people around him to listen to his monologue about his affairs. He dislikes being alone for any length of time.

Holly For the person attacked by thoughts of *jealousy, envy, revenge, suspicion* and *hatred*.

Honeysuckle For one who *dwells upon thoughts of the past*, and is *home-sick*. Such a person does not expect to find in the future the happiness experienced in the past.

Hornbeam For *tiredness, weariness, mental and physical exhaustion*. The person does not have sufficient strength, mentally or physically, to fulfil his work.

Impatiens For he who is quick in thought and action, wishing everything to be done without delay. *Impatient, irritable,* suffering *extreme nervous tension,* this person often has litte patience with others who work more slowly, and prefers to work and think alone.

Larch For *lack of confidence, anticipation of failure* and *despondency*. This person simply does not consider himself as good or capable as those around him, and feels he will never be a success.

Mimulus For the *fears of everyday life*. The *origin of the fear* or anxiety *is known*, and includes illness, pain, fear of being alone, of the dark, of misfortune and accident. The person quietly bears the dread, not talking of it to others.

Mustard For *black depression, melancholia* and *gloom*. Such a person cannot appear happy or cheerful, feeling that a cold, dark cloud overshadows him, hiding the joy of life.

Oak For one who bravely fights on against great difficulties, trying one thing after another in a *never-ceasing effort* to get well or run his affairs better. Often *despondent* and full of *despair* in a hopeless situation, this person never gives up.

Olive For the person who is *completely exhausted* through mental or physical efforts. *Mental fatigue* is such that he feels he has no more strength to make any effort. (Olive is also excellent for exhausted soil, and is often used in vegetable gardens).

Pine — For one who *blames himself*, wallowing in *self-reproach* and *guilt feelings*. *Over-conscientious*, this person is never satisfied with his performance, always thinking he could have done better.

Red Chestnut — For *excessive fear* and *anxiety for others*. This person has often ceased to worry about himself, however, he is overly concerned about others of whom he is fond, anticipating that suffering will descend upon them.

Rock Rose — For *terror* or *extreme fright*, particularly useful in emergencies. The person who is *terrified of travel* should find it valuable.

Rock Water — For the person who is very strict in his way of living: *Repressing himself*, something of a *martyr*, he *denies himself many of the joys and pleasures of life* because they might interfere with his work.

Scleranthus — For *uncertainty, hesitancy* and *changeability of moods*. This person *cannot decide* between two things.

Star of Bethlehem — For the *after-effects of mental or physical shock*, and can be of great comfort to the person who loses someone close, or who has been involved in an accident.

Sweet Chestnut — For those moments when there is *extreme mental anguish*, so great as to appear unbearable. This person feels *hopelessness* and *despair*, as if the mind or body has borne all it can and must now give way.

Vervain — For a *perfectionist* convinced he is right and who wishes to convert other people to his view of life. This person is characterized by *strain, stress, tension, inability to relax*, and over-exertion.

Vine For the *dominating, aggressive, inflexible* and *ambitious* person, certain of his own 'rightness', who wants to persuade others to be like him.

Walnut For *protection from detrimental influence of other people*, as this person may be lead away from his own ideas and aims through the strong opinions of others.

Water Violet For one who is *aloof*, leaving people alone and going his own way. In health and illness, he likes to be left alone. His calmness is a blessing to those around him though his *self-pride* can cause difficulties.

White Chestnut For those who cannot prevent thoughts, ideas, and arguments which they do not desire from entering their minds. These *persistent unwanted thoughts* create *worries* and *mental conversations* which interfere with everyday life.

Wild Oat For *uncertainty, despondence,* and dissatisfaction because one *cannot decide what occupation to follow,* how best to live life. This person *lacks a sense of achievement* for he feels he *has not found his niche in life*.

Wild Rose For one who has given up, is *resigned* to all that happens, *apathetic* and *lacking interest in life*. This person is *embittered for life, resentful* that he has not been treated better. The injustice of life, as he sees it, produces a *negative outlook*.

Willow For those who have suffered adversity and find this difficult to accept without *resentment*. Because they feel they have not deserved so great a trial, they react with *bitterness*. Adopting a *negative outlook* on life, they take less interest in things which they previously enjoyed.

SOME FINAL COMMENTS

From the brief descriptions given above, you will be able to prescribe for yourself and for your family with relative ease. Remember that remedies may be combined to cover the person exhibiting a variety of mental states, and that they may be used for animals and plants as well as for people. Certain remedies have, over the years, proven to be particularly effective and I shall complete this chapter by drawing your attention to them.

In **pregnancy**, as a woman approaches the time of birth, *Mimulus* is of great value in calming the mind and body. *Vervain* and *Impatiens* have also been used effectively to achieve this result. Should fear of childbirth be great, *Rock Rose* may help, and the 'rescue remedy' could well be given a few days before parturition to ease the birth and promote rapid recovery.

For fretful **babies** *Chicory* has often been used very successfully. Should the babies scream for attention, *Impatiens* is likely to soothe them. *Mimulus* can be used if the infant is nervous, frightened of everything, while *Clematis* could be helpful if the baby sleeps too much. It will also be valuable if the infant shows a disinclination to feed, withdrawing into a world of its own and taking no notice of anybody.

With **children**, the more frequently used remedies are *White Chestnut*, when the child broods over problems, beset by constantly recurring negative thoughts; *Agrimony* for those who mask internal misery with a cheerful face; *Willow* for resentments and hatreds; *Holly* for jealousy, envy, rage and suspicion.

Animals injured in accidents show rapid recovery after dosage with the 'rescue remedy'. Should they have ringworm or other skin complaints, *Crab Apple* may bring relief. If driven to distraction by the skin irritation, the animal would probably appreciate *Agrimony*. To strengthen the animal after illness or injury, *Centaury*, *Olive* and *Hornbeam* are all excellent 'revivers'.

As mentioned earlier, *Olive* is valuable in the improvement of impoverished soil. *Vine* and *Wild Oat* serve this purpose also.

For **plants** or trees tortured by blight or any other disease, a combination of *Crab Apple* as a cleanser and *Agrimony* for the torture is likely to bring considerable improvement. Where a tree or plant suffers shock through being transplanted, *Star of Bethlehem* is the remedy to use, followed by *Hornbeam* if its recovery is slow. Alternatively, the 'rescue remedy' could be used. Where plants are weak and droopy, *Centaury*, *Hornbeam* or *Olive* could help as strengtheners. To use the remedies with plants, shrubs or trees, fill a 30-millilitre bottle with rain water and add two drops of the remedy. From this bottle, take 5 ml which is put into 4.5 litres of rain water to make a spray for leaves, branches and roots. With trees, it is necessary to water the ground in a radius equal to the length of the branches in order to reach all the roots.

Speed of response to the remedies varies. Sometimes humans, animals and plants improve with dramatic suddenness after a few doses only. At other times weeks, or even months, might pass before a condition is cured. We have to let nature take its course, aided, in this case, by the Bach remedies. This self-help system of healing has many supporters. Perhaps it will provide the answers to your own ailments and illness. You can only try, knowing you run no risk of damaging yourself in so doing. Should you, after study of each remedy and its description, be unable to arrive at a suitable prescription, try *Wild Oat* or *Holly*, whichever seems closer to your condition. Each of these remedies does seem to have a widely generalized healing effect, and is likely to solve the problem.

6. Schuessler's Biochemic Cell Salts and Your Health

THE SCHUESSLER THEORY

Homoeopathy and the Bach flower remedies are safe, gentle, effective ways of treating your ailments. So, too, is the administration of biochemic cell salts to rectify deficiencies. Dr Wilhelm Schuessler, the originator of this approach to healing, theorizes that the human body contains certain vital inorganic elements which are essential for normal cell function. These elements must be present in physiologically balanced proportion if good health is to be maintained. When one or more of these elements becomes deficient, normal cell function is disturbed and disease is the result. Accordingly, it is necessary to supply to the body, through the blood stream, the inorganic elements which are lacking and thus restore normal physiological balance. These inorganic elements are the *biochemic cell salts* which are twelve in number.

The term 'biochemistry' is derived from the Greek *bios*, meaning life, and 'chemistry' which refers to the chemical changes by which life processes are carried on. These chemical changes are affected by the way in which organic substances unite with inorganic elements to form the different tissues of the body and provide energy for the vital processes of living. When we eat, digest and metabolize healthful foods correctly, inorganic mineral salts such as calcium, potash, sodium, magnesium and phosphorus, pass away from the intestine into the bloodstream. They are thus transported to the specialized cells which need them for survival and health. Each mineral or chemical salt is individually good for specific organs, tissues or body parts. Each has a purpose, so that without cell salts we cannot survive. Our dependence upon them is complete.

As long as we eat sensibly of wholesome food, and our bodies harbour no physical, mental or infectious conflict, we maintain good health. However, if our health circumstances are not so ideal, signs and symptoms of nutritional deficiency show up. Schuessler argues that we must recognize these symptoms and alleviate them with minute doses of the cell salts. Disease occurs, according to his theory, when mineral salts are lacking in the bloodstream and cure comes only when the balance is restored. Therfore, we need to know the twelve biochemic cell salts and the particular symptoms which indicate a deficiency of one or more of them in our system.

THE TWELVE CELL SALTS AND THEIR USES

Calcarea Fluor. (Calcium Fluoride) is found in all elastic fibre, muscular tissues and tooth enamel. Its use is indicated for all ailments involving a relaxed condition of these elastic fibres and the dilation of blood vessels. Thus it can be valuable in the treatment of haemorrhoids, varicose veins, ulcers which affect the bones of the nose, decaying and loose teeth with little enamel, abscesses, goitre, prolapse of the uterus, hard glands, flabby muscles and hiccoughing. *Calcarea Fluor* has also been found of use in cases of blurred vision and cataract.

Calcarea Phos. (Calcium Phosphate) occurs in bone, teeth, blood, connective tissue, the gastric juices and saliva. It gives strength to bone structure, builds firm teeth and forms a valuable part of all secretions of the body. *Calcarea Phos.* has been called 'the great tissue restorer' and has a wide range of uses. It has proven particularly valuable in treating many forms of bone disease, underdevelopment, delayed teething and anaemia, especially of young girls and women. Because it provides a source of quickly utilized calcium it is of use in treating leg cramps, and in promoting rapid healing of bones after fractures. As *Calcarea Phos.* builds new blood corpuscles and restores strength, it can be very helpful if taken during convalescence after illness. Many aches and pains, particularly those which are worse at night and during cold weather yield to this remedy. 'Housemaid's knee' and various rheumatic joint and back pains are of this nature. Gastric disorders, too, seem to be an area of human illness where *Calcarea Phos.* excels as a healing agent, for it relieves gas, colic and diarrhoea as well as alleviating indigestion when food has settled like a heavy weight in the stomach.

Calcarea Sulph. (Calcium Sulphate) is found in the outer layer of the skin, the liver, bile, mucous membranes and the blood. It works to prevent the formation of pus and the disintegration of cells. Accordingly, it is used with suppurative diseases when the discharge is thick, yellow and bloody. Wounds discharging pus, skin ailments with yellow scabs, pimples discharging blood and pus, catarrh with thick yellow mucus are all likely to yield to *Calcarea Sulph.* It is excellent with skin disease and where any part of the body shows discharge for a period of time without healing. Other illnesses for which this tissue salt may be used are tonsillitis, croup, and disorders of elimination such as diarrhoea or constipation. The main way to judge whether this remedy is the one you need is to observe whether eruptions come to a head. If they do, *Calcarea Sulph.* is likely to promote healing for you.

Ferrum Phos. (Iron Phosphate) is present in the blood, helping to form red corpuscles and carry oxygen throughout the body. This remedy is particularly valuable for fever, inflammation and congestive disease, so bronchitis, sore throats, coughs, colds, rheumatism, bladder and kidney irritations and congestive headaches are all likely to yield to its healing effects. When anaemia is due to a lack of red corpuscles, *Ferrum Phos.* can be very helpful, as it can when a person suffers haemorrhages from any part of the body. In addition to hastening the healing of inflammations and haemorrhages, these iron salts promote recovery from contusions, discolorations and sprains so it is a valuable remedy for the sportsman and sportswoman.

Kali Mur. (Potassium Chloride) unites with albumen to form filarin which is present in every tissue of the body. Should this cell salt be lacking, no new brain cell formation would occur.

Indication of a deficiency of *Kali Mur.* is a thick white discharge from mucous surfaces and a whitish grey coating on the tongue. Other indications are stomach upsets due to eating rich or fatty foods and hurts being aggravated by motion. Uses of *Kali Mur.* include croup, dysentery, catarrh of nose, throat and other organs when the usual white discharge is present, rheumatism, skin disease with eruption of white matter, mumps and whooping cough. It has also been used to treat asthma, though I would suggest *Kali Phos.* as a remedy of first choice for this illness. Another use to which this remedy has been put is for the dissolving of blood clots, and it has been suggested that a person who suffers a stroke should be given *Kali Mur.* as soon as possible.

Kali Phos. (Potassium Phosphate) is a constituent of brain, nerves, muscles and blood, and a deficiency results in mental and nervous disorders. It is, accordingly, of great value in ailments such as loss of memory, prostration, brain fag, nervous headaches and those brought on by mental overstrain, all neuralgia pains, general debility and exhaustion, sleeplessness from nervous causes, nervous indigestion, hysteria, heart palpitations and general depression. As the 'great nerve remedy' *Kali Phos.* helps people overcome a loss of personal drive, and is of particular benefit with the weepy, suspicious patient. Respiratory problems generally, and asthma in particular, if it has nervous manifestation, are likely to benefit from treatment with *Kali Phos.* It has been used with success to treat inability to retain urine, muscle spasms, carbuncles, and stomach ulcers. There is evidence that this remedy acts as an antiseptic in the body and halts decay, though its main function is as a neutralizer of nervous distress and neurasthenia.

Kali Sulph. (Potassium Sulphate) is found in the outer skin layer and in skin cells. It acts as an oxygen carrier and is vital to normal functioning of the glands and for regulation of the quantity of water in the tissues. A deficiency of this cell salt is indicated by yellowish, watery secretions and a yellow coated tongue. If you lack *Kali Sulph.* you are likely to feel chilly, experience dizziness, toothache, headaches, and pain in your hands and feet. These problems become worse towards evening and during warm weather, but are relieved by coolness and being out in the open air. *Kali Sulph.* has been used successfully for catarrh of the nose, throat, stomach and urinary organs, coughs, bronchitis, eye diseases with a slimy discharge, delayed menstruation, measles and chicken pox. It can be quite valuable, also, in the treatment of rashes.

Magnesia Phos. (Magnesia Phosphate) occurs in the brain and in the white fibres of nerves and muscles. A deficiency often shows up as spasms, cramps and convulsions as the fibres contract. The use of *Magnesia Phos.* are many and varied, including the treatment of shooting, boring, nagging points which change their position frequently, all forms of spasm, especially back pain which comes in spasms, neuralgia of the face and head, such as earache, toothache, headache, stomach cramps, asthma with a convulsive cough, all types of cramps, angina pectoris, diarrhoea, menstrual colic, spasmodic retention of urine and acute neuritis. It is worth remembering that this remedy works more quickly if it is taken in hot water.

Natrum Mur. (Sodium Chloride), or common table salt, is found in combination with water throughout the living cells, regulating the amount of moisture present in all body parts and ensuring a correct proportion of water in the body fluids. Indication of deficiency lies primarily in the presence of thin, watery discharges, symptoms including anaemia, asthma mucus, bronchitis phlegm, hay fever and eczema. *Natrum Mur.* is used to treat aches of all kinds, such as headache and stomach ache, constipation, excessive salivation, vomiting of water and mucous, watery diarrhoea, skin diseases with watery discharges, and indigestion with watery vomiting.

Natrum Phos. (Sodium Phosphate), when present in the blood, muscles, nerves, brain and intercellular fluids, regulates digestion and neutralizes the formation of waste lactic acid. If there is a lack of this cell salt, there is an excess of acid in the system. This reveals itself in an acid condition of the stomach with sour vomiting, sour stools, colic spasm and fever, and in complaints such as rheumatism, arthritis and gout.

Accordingly, *Natrum Phos.* may be used to treat these complaints, particularly acute arthritis and gout, for it acts to dissolve uric acid around the joints. Possibly the best indication for its use is the presence of a tongue-coated golden yellow, together with the excess gastric acidity already mentioned. When a golden yellow secretion is present with eczema or inflamed eyes, it is a strong indication that *Natrum Phos.* lacking in the system, and improved health is likely to result from remedying this deficiency. As it is basically an antidote to acidity and sourness, *Natrum Phos.* is valuable in cases of heart burn and sour smelling perspiration. Urinary tract disorders such as gravel, may also respond well to this remedy.

Natrum Sulph. (Sodium Sulphate), Glauber's Salt, is present in the intercellular fluids, regulating the quantity of water in body tissues and the blood. Its other main function is to assist in keeping bile at its correct consistency, and a strong indication for its use is when you become conscious of an excess of bile in your system. Signs of this include a dirty brown or greyish green coating of the tongue, a bitter taste in the mouth, intermittent fever with vomiting of bile, and bilious sick headaches. These symptoms are usually relieved when *Natrum Sulph.* is taken, as are diarrhoea, gallstones, dizziness, vomiting during pregnancy, influenza headache, jaundice and congestion of the liver. Skin diseases which have bilious symptoms yield to this remedy as does gout, for it is an excellent antidote for excess uric acid in the system. Considerable success has also been reported by people using *Natrum Sulph.* to reduce blood pressure. It is worth bearing in mind, too, that this remedy has proven of great value for people living in damp places who suffer from muscle and joint pain.

Silicea is present in connective tissue, skin, hair and nails, and has a considerable reputation as an agent for conquering infection. It controls suppuration by bringing boils, carbuncles, ulcers and abscesses to a head, and is particularly prized in the treatment of a wide range of skin problems. Discharges of thick yellow pus are an indication for its use, but its application is not limited to the treatment of such problems. *Silicea* can be employed to treat chronic nasal catarrh, bone problems, gout, and to relieve arthritic pain. One of its actions is to help muscles relax and to aid in the absorption of blood from injuries. Thus, it has been found useful in the treatment of sports injuries such as sprains and, together with *Calcarea Phos.*, has often relieved the discomfort and disfiguration of a 'black eye'. Another eye problem, that of thick offensive discharges and secretions, also calls for use of this remedy.

SELF-TREATMENT OF CELL SALT DEFICIENCIES

It has been frequently suggested that cell salt deficiencies are often a function of our use of over-refined modern foods. Normally, we would expect to derive all the necessary constituents of a healthy body from the food we eat, but this presupposes that processing has not removed these constituents. For example, during refinement, bread made from wheaten flour is stripped of many essential salts and minerals. Cooking, too, may often rob foods of these salts and a condition of mineral deficiency becomes apparent.

Robert Hill, the son of a colleague of mine, revealed the typical symptoms of a body starved of mineral cell salts. He seemed listless, apathetic and depressed. Each evening he literally dragged himself home from his job as a bank teller, apparently lacking energy and interest in life. At night, though very tired, he was often unable to sleep. In addition, he was troubled with nervous indigestion, neuralgia and constant headaches. *Kali Phos.*, one of the twelve biochemic cell salts, was the remedy Robert took to help him back to health.

He arrived at this remedy through his own reading, after three different doctors were unable to do anything for him. Actually, as mentioned earlier, each cell salt has a very clearly defined action, and *Kali Phos.* usually helps people with 'nerves'. Robert found he was sleeping better, his appetite improved, his skin took on a healthier appearance, his nervous indigestion and headaches abated, and generally his brightness and energy re-appeared. These gains were achieved by allowing tablets of *Kali Phos.* to dissolve in the saliva of his mouth from whence the cell salt was carried by the blood stream directly to the diseased tissue, thus enabling 'healing' to commence immediately.

Robert's recovery was quite rapid, three weeks in all, but it is often difficult to predict how quickly the administration of cell salts will effect a cure. Sometimes only days are needed if corrective treatment is begun immediately the symptoms show themselves. In other cases, particularly when the illness has been present for some time, months may be needed before there is a return to normal health.

According to Schuessler, then, every tiny cell is specialized in its own way. Every organ and body part contains these cells and their total health is determined by incredibly small particles of minerals or biochemic salts that feed them. When health fails, diagnose your symptoms and prescribe the appropriate cell salt to rectify the deficiency. Again, as with homoeopathy and the Bach remedies, the secret of administration lies in a minimum dose of a substance which is completely harmless, drug-free, and able to be given with perfect safety to the youngest child.

Schuessler, like Hahnemann and Bach, has developed a system of self-help 'medicine'. We read many warnings from eminent medical authorities about the dangers of treating ourselves—and sometimes they are right. Not always, though. As Dr W. E. Shute has commented in his book *Vitamin E for Ailing and Healthy Hearts:* Of course people shouldn't treat themselves [but] . . . fortunately the average patient has more to gain by treating himself than he has to lose by poor selection of a doctor.'

With treatment methods such as homoeopathy, the Bach remedies, and Schuessler's cell salts, the risks from self-treatment are minimal. If the selected remedy does not help you, it is most unlikely to harm you. Can the same be said for the drugs prescribed, perhaps incorrectly, by a less than competent doctor? Should you choose your doctor well, you will normally escape harm, but what medical authorities consistently overlook when they warn against self-help medicine is that some doctors not only do not help their patients, but, inadvertently, cause them harm through the drugs they prescribe.

GENERAL PRINCIPLES OF SELF-PRESCRIPTION

In his *Handbook of Unusual and Unorthodox Healing Methods*, Cerney has provided useful summary statements as guides to selection of the appropriate biochemic cell salt. Taking an overall view:

- The Phosphates (*Calcarea Phos.*, *Ferrum Phos.*, *Kali Phos.*, *Magnesia Phos.*, *Natrum Phos.*,) are primarily remedies for problems of the nervous system and for the treatment of muscles.
- The Chlorides (*Kali Mur.*, *Natrum Mur.*,) are primarily for muscle problems.
- The Sulphates (*Calcarea Sulph.*, *Kali Sulph.*, *Natrum Sulph.*,) are primarily for the treatment of bone problems.

This is, of course, a very general categorization. It is necessary to learn the particular characteristics of each remedy and to ascertain your own specific signs and symptoms before you can use Schuessler's system of self-help therapy. If you have inflammation in some body part, a sore throat for example, *Ferrum Phos.* is likely to be the remedy of choice. However, should you experience soreness without accompanying inflammation, *Natrum Phos.*, is more likely to effect the cure you seek. This less general approach to self-diagnosis may be set out in the following way:

General symptom	Cell salt to use
Inflammation	*Ferrum Phos.*
Soreness and acidity	*Natrum Sulph.*
Pain	*Magnesia Phos.*
Low temperature making pain worse	*Calcarea Phos.*

Fever or soreness after exercise	Kali Phos., Natrum Phos.
Problems worsened by warmth and improved by coldness. All discharges yellow in colour.	Kali Sulph.
Muscle spasms, cramps, pain relieved by warmth and pressure.	Magnesia Phos., Calcarea Phos., Silicea
Croupy cough, dental problems, bulging varicose veins.	Calcarea Fluor.
All bilious problems	Natrum Sulph.
Greyish white secretions on tongue.	Kali Mur.
Symptoms made worse by motion.	Kali Mur.

Use of this table can provide a quick reference for matching the appropriate tissue salt with your symptoms. However, it is then desirable to use the more detailed description of the twelve salts given earlier in this chapter.

DOSAGE

A study of the twelve cell salts should enable you to prescribe the remedy most appropriate to your symptoms with relative ease. However, the question of dosage remains. As with homoeopathy and the Bach remedies, this does not seem critical. Because of the harmless nature of the substances used, overdosing produces no adverse side effects. On the other hand, neither does it produce benefits over and above those gained through administration of the minimal dose.

Probably the most commonly used unit is the large 7.5 gram tablet which is obtainable from homoeopaths, naturopaths and, sometimes, health stores, in 3X, 6X or 12X potency. Suggested dosage for adults would be one of these tablets taken four times a day, before meals and at bedtime. Children would follow the same dosage pattern with half a tablet as would babies, though their dose would be further reduced to quarter of a tablet four times a day. These tablets are normally taken dry, dissolving on or under the tongue, or crushed and chewed in the mouth without water to wash them down. This is because cell salts are not assimilated in the digestive tract but are absorbed directly through the tissues.

In cases of severe pain, this mode of administration may be varied so that the remedies are given in hot water which increases the speed of their action. When such pain is present, or with acute diseases generally, doses may be given every quarter or half-hour. Where the case is less urgent, tablets may be taken every one or two hours. As with homoeopathic remedies, discontinue the treatment once improvement becomes noticeable. Should this improvement cease, resume taking the remedy.

FOOD: MINERAL SALTS IN THEIR NATURAL FORM

Ingrid Sherman, in her book *Natural Remedies*, has listed each of the twelve biochemic cell salts with the foods, primarily vegetables and fruit, in which they are found. Some readers may prefer to absorb their tissue salts in this way rather than in tablet form. The problem is, should deficiencies show up, it is difficult to control the dosage. However, ensuring an adequate supply of the essential tissue salts through a judicious choice of vegetables and fruit is preventive medicine at its best, for you thus protect yourself against such deficiencies.

Among the vegetables, **lettuce**, (*Calc. Fluor., Calc. Phos., Ferrum Phos., Kali Phos., Kali Sulph., Magnesia Phos., Natrum Mur.,*) **spinach** (*Calc. Phos., Ferrum Phos., Kali Mur., Kali Phos., Natrum Phos., Natrum Mur., Natrum Sulph.,*) and **cucumber** (*Calc. Phos., Ferrum Phos., Kali Phos., Kali Sulph., Magnesia Phos., Natrum Mur., Natrum Sulph.*) are particularly valuable, each of them containing seven of the twelve cell salts. Other vegetables which are almost as good are **cabbage** (six salts), **asparagus** (six salts), **onions** (five salts), and **radishes** (five salts).

Figs (*Calc. Phos., Calc. Sulph., Magnesia Phos., Natrum Mur.,*

Natrum Phos., Silicea) and **strawberries** *(Calc. Phos., Calc. Sulph., Ferrum Phos., Natrum Sulph., Silicea)* contain six of the cell salts and are possibly the richest of the fruits in this respect. However, **apples** with five salts and **blueberries** with four are also very valuable.

Other good food sources of the mineral salts are **almonds** (five salts), **coconuts** (four salts) and **whole wheat** (four salts). For readers who require more detailed information on exactly which foods contain which cell salts, I strongly recommend Sherman's book. As well as giving this information about the Schuessler therapy, it contains much worthwhile advice on improving your health through the use of natural remedies.

AN OVERABUNDANCE OF RICHES

The Schuessler cell salts, Bach's flower remedies, and Hahnemann's homoeopathic remedies surely provide an abundance of natural, safe remedies. Abundance, however, provides its own problems, one of which is choice. Confronted by so many remedies which purport to 'cure' the same ailments, how is one to choose among them? Where do we start? In each of the last four chapters I have tried to provide a guide to help you in your decisions but this may not be sufficient. There is an alternative, however, which might appeal to you, one which appears to make use of unconscious mental processes instead of relying completely on conscious, rational decision making. We'll consider it in the next chapter.

7. Dowsing for Improved Health

THE PENDULUM

In an earlier book, *The Plus Factor: a guide to positive living*, I outlined the process of dowsing as a method of taking the strain out of decision making. A pendulum, consisting of a weight or bob suspended by a thread or a fine chain, may be used in this process. It can take any form, as long as it can be held comfortably and swing freely. A length of about 10 cm is convenient to work with, while the weight may be virtually any material, such as wood, glass, plastic, crystal or metal. As with length of thread and composition of the bob, weight is a matter of personal preference. However, should you wish to use the pendulum with lists or charts, two methods which will be presently described, it is desirable for the weight to be pointed at the bottom. A teardrop shape, for example, would be of value in this context. Should you wish to use a pendulum which is not so shaped, I suggest you heat a needle and push it into the bottom of the weight. If the material of your bob makes this impossible, a pin could be stuck to the bottom of the pendulum with glue.

Four basic reactions are available from the pendulum. One is a to-and-fro oscillation towards and away from you. Another is a back-and-forth oscillation across your body from left to right and from right to left. A third is a rotary movement in a clockwise direction while a fourth reverses this rotation so that an anti-clockwise movement is observable. It is these movements which provide the answers to the questions which you ask, but there is no 'right' interpretation. You need to find out, by trial and error, what each movement means for you. Simply because oscillation across my body means 'yes' for me and oscillation towards and away from my body means 'no', it does not follow that you will obtain the same reaction. For you, 'yes' might be a clockwise rotation and 'no' an anticlockwise rotation.

Perhaps the simplest way of establishing what meaning each movement has for you is the following. Suspend the pendulum by its thread, bending your elbow so your forearm is approximately parallel with the ground. If you so desire, you may support your elbow on a table or chair arm. Now, focus your attention on the pendulum bob and think 'yes'. If no movement develops after, say thirty or forty seconds, vary the length of the thread, either letting it run through your fingers to lengthen it, or wrapping more around your fingers to shorten it. You will 'know' the 'right' length for you—it feels comfortable and the pendulum bob moves about smoothly. Once you have established your 'yes' or positive direction, think 'no'. As you focus your mind on this negative statement you'll find your pendulum moving in a different way. The other two possible directions will be responses to you focussing your mind upon two more statements, firstly 'I don't know', and secondly 'I don't want to tell you'.

When I first commenced using the pendulum for decision making I believed all four movements were necessary. I no longer do. You need only your 'yes' and 'no' responses. If you get a response which is neither 'yes' nor 'no', I would suggest that you have phrased your question poorly and a rewording will provide a definite positive or a definite negative answer. The manner in which you word your questions is critical. You must be quite clear what you want to ask the pendulum and phrase this query in unambiguous terms. Then, be sure you remember exactly how you worded your question so that you can interpret the answer clearly.

To illustrate, let us imagine your car is two-toned, cream and brown. You ask your pendulum: 'Is this car blue in colour?' and you should get a 'no' answer. You then ask: 'Is this car brown in colour?' In this case, you are likely to get an 'I don't know' response because both 'yes' and 'no' would be incorrect answers. In fact, what is really being indicated in such an answer is both 'yes' and 'no'. Rephrasing of the question to 'Is one of the colours of this car brown?' will bring you a 'yes' response. Perhaps this is a trite example but it does illustrate the point that questions must be clearly stated if 'I don't know' type responses are to be avoided. Vaguely formulated questions bring vague answers, a reason why people reject the pendulum as a useful decision making device. It is not the tool, that is, the pendulum, which is normally at fault, but the person using it.

YOUR BELIEF SYSTEM

One of the reasons a person may get no response from a pendulum is his belief system. If he dismisses the whole idea as rubbish, he is virtually giving a directive to his subconscious mind to do nothing. However, should a person believe that the pendulum will work for him, he is likely to attain instant success. This is true whether he believes the 'official' theory of why the pendulum works, whether he has an explanation of his own, or whether he has a simple faith because he has been told, or read about, the success of others with this device.

The 'official' theory is that the pendulum is a way of establishing a channel to the subconscious mind which, it is suggested, contains the record of everything which has happened to us since the moment of our birth. If you can accept the subconscious mind as a repository of your life's experiences, then obviously it must know more about you than your conscious mind. Thus, it is in a better position to advise you on making decisions, as I've outlined in *The Plus Factor*, and on improving your health, which is the context of this present book. Because the subconscious mind can produce involuntary muscle movements, it can be taught to move a pendulum and thereby speak directly to the conscious mind.

The subconscious mind, therefore, by means of the pendulum, provides data to the conscious mind, which then observes and interprets this data. There is no special power in the pendulum as such. It is only an instrumental aid helping you to focus your mind upon a particular question to which you require an answer. Because it presumably taps deeper knowledge than that contained in the conscious mind, it is likely to give you a better answer than that obtainable by normal conscious processes.

If you can believe this explanation of how the pendulum functions, well and good, for this belief will virtually ensure that it works. However, the main thing is to keep an open mind and realize that dowsing is a relatively simple, straight-forward process. Do not complicate it by believing in the need for special requirements to make the pendulum move, for once you do, your pendulum will not work unless these requirements are present.

John Pearse, for example, read that his pendulum should contain a drop of his blood to make 'the vibrations compatible'. As long as John consciously thought his pendulum contained the drop of blood, it worked beautifully for him. Other pendulums remained motionless for him because he believed that they were 'incompatible' with him. However, on one occasion, a duplicate of John's instrument, lacking only the blood drop, was substituted without his knowledge. Naturally it worked perfectly. It is the conscious mind which must advise the subconscious that the requirement has not been met. When it does receive such an instruction, it obediently fails to direct the appropriate muscle movement.

Similarly if you are taught, or read, that a certain length of thread is necessary, or your bob must be a certain weight, or the composition of your pendulum must be a certain material, and you believe these things, your dowsing becomes a prisoner of your beliefs. These exert a limiting influence. If you restrict your dowsing activities, as many people do, to a certain time of the day, or when the 'aura is right', or when the weather is appropriate, you have established certain limitations from which you will find it difficult to escape.

This process of limitation through beliefs is part of the wider issue I touch on repeatedly throughout this book. We live not with things, objects, but with ideas about things. It is the labels we place upon those objects, and our emotions and prejudices which get in our way and stop us making use of our full potential. This is because our ideas about things prevent us seeing the things themselves. Science, physics, law, religion, psychiatry and economics are all frameworks which try to organize reality, by providing ideas about the way life is. But they are only ideas about life, not absolute truths.

We come back, then, to the basic theme of trying things out for yourself, of trying out the pendulum to find if it will help you select remedies which will improve your health. The great mistake is to try and learn how to dowse by reading about or talking about it instead of doing it. You can become very confused by the conflicting statements emanating from different people all of whom might be able to use the pendulum successfully. These people do not really know why it works for them—it just does. So practise first, then maybe you can arrive at an explanation of what has happened which will satisfy you. Like any other human activity, practice is the key. The more you use your pendulum the sooner you gain the required ability and confidence.

SOME PENDULUM EXERCISES

To become familiar with the use of the pendulum, it is desirable to measure or evaluate things which will not create important problems if you are wrong. As you sharpen your questioning skill and check out the answers the pendulum provides, you will gain confidence in the data it can provide for you, and feel comfortable in using it to make decisions about your health. It is best not to rush into pendulum prescribing, however, until you do attain this confidence. The following or similar exercises should enable you to do so in an enjoyable way.

An avid reader and film goer, Alan Stephenson used his pendulum as a predictive instrument. Before he started a new book, or saw a film, he would ask whether he was likely to enjoy it or not. He would then read the book, or see the film, deciding on a 'yes/no' basis whether he had actually enjoyed it or not. No great harm was done if the pendulum predictions proved to be wrong, for in his 'experiments', Alan used only books he intended to read and films he intended to see. Thus, this 'exercise' provided a non-risk practice area, one which quickly built up Alan's confidence in his pendulum answers for they proved a very accurate guide.

Jenni Sturgess went about her practice a different way. She found it difficult to accept the idea that the pendulum provided a means of communication with an all-wise subconscious mind, and preferred not to start with 'yes/no' responses. Instead she wanted to find whether the pendulum would actually move for her without her asking direct questions. What she did was to sit comfortably at a table on which was placed a sheet of white paper. On this paper, she put a pencil. Holding the pendulum lightly between her thumb and forefinger, Jenni held it over the middle of the pencil. Her arm was relaxed and her elbow rested on the table for support. Because of her scepticism, Jenni was not really expecting anything particular to happen. However, she was sufficiently open-minded to be reasonably neutral, adopting a receptive 'wait-and-see' attitude. In fact, she imagined herself as a supersensitive receiving set waiting to pick up any incoming signals, an excellent state of mind to adopt for this work.

After a short time, the pendulum began oscillating along the length of the pencil. As a reasonable swing built up, Jenni slowly moved the pendulum towards the tip of the pencil, at which point the movement changed from oscillation to a clockwise rotation. As she moved her hand back from the tip, the oscillation recommenced, changing to an anti-clockwise rotation when the other end of the pencil was reached.

Jenni's experience provides a useful guide for those of you who want to test your dowsing ability. She did not make up her mind about the results she wanted. She simply waited patiently, giving the pendulum time to work. Often it takes up to half a minute or even more before movement commences, though usually only a few seconds is necessary. If you try Jenni's pencil exercise, do not expect to get the same reactions as she did. You might — but then again you might not. However, as far as Jenni was concerned, she had demonstrated that the pendulum would move, seemingly of its own accord without her willing it to do so.

A point to keep in mind with exercises such as this is to do them for a brief period only. With longer practice sessions, it can become a temptation to exert conscious control over the pendulum movement and produce confused results. However, should you so desire, you can repeat the experiment at frequent intervals, say each day, until the pendulum reactions occur more rapidly. This is most likely if you practise alone, at least until you have developed confidence in your use of the instrument.

Bill Evans is a card player. Naturally enough, his familiarization exercises with the pendulum involved using cards. He would select, say, three red cards and one black, shuffle them thoroughly, place them face downward on a table and ask his pendulum to indicate which was the black card by giving a 'yes' answer. An interesting exercise this, but one which does not seem to bear repetition too frequently. Many people get quite accurate results initially, but then the pendulum answers become increasingly inaccurate. It is difficult to understand why this should be so, but experienced dowsers warn against repetition which seems to confuse the dowsing faculty. First readings would appear to be most reliable if the mind is clear and the question precisely worded. However, if this first reading leaves the pendulum user in some doubt, he is often inclined to repeat the procedure several times. A preferable strategy would be to reframe the question coming at it from a different angle. Should inconsistency or lack of clarity continue, readings are of doubtful value and it would be advisable to postpone further work until another time.

An English midwife, Betty Turner, used to amuse herself and her expectant mothers by predicting the sex of their unborn babies by noting the movement of the pendulum. This 'exercise' has been a popular one for years and Betty, along with many other people, can verify that correctness of prediction far exceeds that which would be expected by chance. Either the conventional 'yes/no' procedure can be followed, asking 'Is the baby female?' or simply, through experience, noting that the pendulum always tends to swing in the same way for females, usually anti-clockwise, and for males, usually clockwise. You can test this on your friends and the consistency of the results you obtain will increase your confidence in the pendulum's answers.

If you enjoy figures you might like to try the exercise of working out a number of mathematical calculations on separate pieces of paper. In some of these calculations make deliberate errors. With the pieces of paper face downward on a table, suspend your pendulum over each one asking whether the calculation is correct. On one occasion, when a friend of mine tried this, he found the pendulum to be incorrect only once out of a dozen tries. It claimed one of his correct calculations was incorrect. Interestingly enough, when he checked it, he found he was wrong and the pendulum was right, for he had made an error without meaning to do so. When things like this happen, it does offer some support for the theory that the pendulum is tapping the vaster knowledge of the subconscious mind.

A final exercise, this time involving a test of water purity may interest you. Have someone fill half a dozen cups with tap water and put a tablespoon of salt in one of these. Naturally, you are kept in ignorance of which cup has been so treated and must rely on the pendulum to identify the salty water. Again, this exercise is likely to work only once at any particular time, but can be repeated on different occasions.

PSYCHOLOGICAL INTERFERENCE

As a result of the practice you do with your pendulum, you will learn something of your ability as a dowser. However, as with most of our activities, it is often the obstacles we create in our own minds which interfere with our success. In his book, *Dowsing*, Tom Graves uses psychological interference as a general term to cover a range of problems all of which involve the intrusion of the mind into the dowsing process.

The first of these is *our attempt to consciously control the process*. We seem to be unwilling to trust subconscious, intuitive processes, feeling we must impose our conscious rationality upon decision making. Yet, pause to reflect how often your rationally arrived at decisions have proven to be quite wrong, and how often your intuitive flashes have proven correct. Both conscious and subconscious processes are of value, but if you are using a method which attempts to tap subconscious information, keep the conscious mind from interfering. Avoid confusing the mind with contradictory orders. Allow the pendulum to operate 'as if' it has a life and mind of its own. This may seem a rather peculiar attitude to take, but by allowing the instrument an existence independent of your conscious control, you permit it to operate more effectively.

A second problem involves the *intrusion of conscious and semiconscious assumptions*, and the associated problem of failing to keep your mind on what you are supposed to be doing. It is a matter of balance, really, focussing your awareness on the question you are asking without allowing your assumptions to interfere with the pendulum's answering procedure. Be aware of simple slips like: 'Last time I asked this sort of question I got this response, so I should get it again.'

However, it is the third problem, that of the *unconscious intrusion of assumptions and prejudices*, which can be most damaging. To guard against such intrusion, it seems necessary to isolate yourself from the process as far as possible. Obviously the part of you which is posing the question must be involved, but otherwise you act as an onlooker, an observer. Experienced meditators can, for example, use the pendulum while resting in a meditative state. For non-meditators, Graves suggests that, when dowsing, you rest your mind on the balance of the pendulum, on where you are, and on the problem at hand. By so doing you avoid the common errors of trying to get a result, doubting your ability to get answers, and trying to prove something. All these are states of mind which are obstacles to effective pendulum usage. Let it work for you and forget about trying to prove to someone else that it works.

It is helpful to direct your attention to your instrument and away from your hands. This leads to adoption of a more disinterested observer stance, and is something akin to the distraction of attention technique which can work so well at the dentist's. Instead of concentrating on yourself, and your reactions to the injection, the drill, and the various instruments the dentist uses, you could do well to focus on the dentist and what *he* is doing. By directing your attention in this way you are likely to reduce your anxiety and your discomfort.

THE PENDULUM AND CHOOSING A REMEDY

Assuming you have tried various exercises, have developed some confidence in your dowsing ability, and have established a definite pendulum movement for 'yes' and 'no', you are in a position to use this approach for the purpose of choosing a suitable remedy. As previous chapters have described homoeopathy, the Bach remedies and the Schuessler cell salts, I'll use an example based on this self-help approach to healing.

In homoeopathic diagnosis, the idea is to find the *similimum*, the substance which, given in a large dose, would create symptoms in a healthy person closely matching those symptoms exhibited by the patient. Dowsing can be helpful in the indentification of this *similimum*: first, by checking the description of symptoms given by the patient, second, by selecting from the remedies given in the homoeopathic *Materia Medica* the one most likely to prove best for that particular ill person at that particular time, and third, by finding the correct potency and dosage.

Now, we may know what remedies might be of value to us should we fall ill or injure ourselves, but sometimes we are uncertain which one is likely to be most suited to the nature of our problem. It is in such a situation that the pendulum might be used to make the choice. There are several ways in which this may be done. You might take one of these remedies at a time, in your pendulum hand, and hold it over the injured area. Should it be the appropriate one, the pendulum will give a positive or 'yes' response. Alternatively, you may prefer to hold the remedy in your free hand.

In both the above cases, the actual bottles containing the 'medicine' are used, but this is not really necessary. Instead, while holding your pendulum over the injured area, you could point with the forefinger of your free hand either to the bottle or to the name of the remedy written on a list. That is, you work down the list, pointing to each preparation in turn until you receive a positive response. Sometimes charts may be used instead of lists and an example of this approach will be described later in the chapter. Actually, none of these physical aids is essential, for merely by thinking of one remedy at a time, you can make your choice. Bottles, lists and charts are useful devices for focussing the mind and if you believe they help you, they will do so. However, many people select their remedies by asking: 'Is *Arnica* (or *Rhus tox.* or *Ruta*) the right remedy?' while holding their pendulum over the injury.

Once the appropriate remedy has been identified you can ask: 'Should this remedy be administered at ∅ (or 6X or 12X) potency?' This is, of course, for remedies taken internally. External remedies are applied as lotions or ointments as explained in Chapters 3 and 4.

Potencies in general use range from the mother tincture, ∅, through 1X, 2X, 3X, 6X, 12X, 30X to 200X. I would suggest, however, that you make 12X your top limit as there have been some reports of adverse effects produced by incorrect prescribing of remedies at the 30X and 200X levels. Finally, you inquire of your pendulum the frequency of dosage required or, if it is external remedy, of application. This answer should be checked as the injury improves, for a patient's requirements change as his condition changes.

Selection of the appropriate remedy, whether it be a homoeopathic preparation, a Bach preparation, or a cell salt, may be achieved in the way outlined above. The same method can be used with proprietary medicines available from pharmacies. If your pendulum gives a positive response, you can feel more confident in taking such medicines.

Also, by dowsing, you can ascertain when the medicine is no longer required, or whether a change should be made. After taking the medicine for several days, perhaps no improvement in your condition is apparent. In this case, it might be worthwhile asking your pendulum if the remedy is actually assisting your body to heal itself. If the answer is 'no', you could then think of possible alternatives, selecting from among them in the way already outlined. However, use of the pendulum to make a choice among possible remedies is only one way of dowsing for improved health. There are others.

THE CONCEPT OF HARMONY

A healthy body is a harmonious body with all its systems interacting with each other smoothly. This is internal harmony. External harmony sees the healthy body relating effectively with the outside world so that there is no excessive stress. To help us maintain such a state, we can test the food we eat and the fluid we drink to ascertain whether they are harmonious to us, whether they are likely to improve our health or likely to damage it. The usual 'yes/no' system can serve this purpose.

Should we get a 'no' response, then we will have to find out why. Graves, to whom I referred earlier, suggests we ask questions such as: 'Is there too much food there? Or too much drink? Is one particular part of the meal damaging? Is it overcooked?' Another useful query is: 'Has this food been prepared in aluminium utensils?' Many people are allergic to aluminium, and aluminium absorption can be very detrimental to health. Actually, you can test your reaction by boiling up some water in an aluminium kettle or saucepan and pouring some of it into a cup. This can then be tested as you would any article of diet with the question: 'Is this water damaging to my health?'

Whether a particular item of food is good for you can also be tested by suspending your pendulum over the back of your hand until it establishes the movement characteristic of you. Then slowly move you hand over the food. Should the swing remain constant, it would appear you and the food are in harmony. Any change in swing would suggest a disharmony which should be tracked down by asking specific questions as described above. Another way of achieving the same end is to point the forefinger of your free hand towards the particular article of food, asking whether it is in harmony with you.

Of course, all this can be greatly overdone. We do tend to get carried away by fads and can finish up too worried to eat anything. In fact, if you practise on the things you eat and drink for a month you can probably forget about doing it any further as you'll know simply by looking at something whether it is good for you or not. Pendulum practice does seem to sharpen our judgements in this way.

Jan Ferguson found this to be true. For several weeks she pendulum-tested everything she took from her refrigerator to ascertain whether it had been stored there too long. However, after this period she checked only occasionally as her previous, often incorrect, judgement had improved considerably. What really happened with Jan is that she developed more confidence in her own diagnostic ability through using the pendulum. Initially though, she was very doubtful about her likely success as a dowser.

This is definitely a problem with pendulum analysis. How do you know whether you have sufficient skill to achieve reasonable accuracy and beneficial results? Doing the exercises described earlier in this chapter is one way of finding out. Another, suggested by Finch in *The Pendulum and Your Health*, is to start with household plants, employing a pendulum to determine their needs for nutrients and moisture. You can check on the accuracy of your analysis by the condition of the plant—does it thrive or not? Use the pendulum to determine which of the plant foods available is best for particular plants, and in what quantities it should be administered. Discover the amount of water required for optimum growth. Test soil and water for harmful content. Learn whether a change of potting material is necessary. By the time you have practiced in this way on your plants and those of your acquaintances, you will know whether you have the skill to improve your own health through pendulum analysis.

ADVANCED PENDULUM DIAGNOSIS

Many people use the pendulum as a diagnostic instrument,

though such diagnosis is usually restricted to minor ailments. This is an intelligent way to use dowsing for it is certainly not infallible. Like any other method of diagnosis, it is right sometimes and wrong sometimes. If you suspect your problem is serious, obviously a medical opinion is helpful. Although I have, in previous chapters, been talking about supplements and alternatives to traditional medicine, I would not suggest an outright rejection of such treatment. Often it is the *only* known curative agent for a particular disease. Frequently it is the *best* treatment among those available.

Where the pendulum can be more useful, however, is in the minor ailments which plague our daily existence, or with those vague symptoms which conventional medicine finds so difficult to treat. When you are not enjoying the buoyant health you desire, all possible avenues should be explored for means of improvement. Include traditional medicine in your search but realize it is not the only path. Through use of the pendulum, you may be able to arrive at a health regime best for you, one which your doctor may not have been able to prescribe for you.

The pendulum can detect faults in the human or animal body. You can prove this to yourself quite simply. Hold your pendulum over the back of your free hand. You should obtain a positive or 'yes' reaction indicating healthy tissue. I am assuming here that your hand is healthy, that you are not suffering from skin trouble or tissue damage in this area. Now slap the back of your hand smartly, and try the pendulum again. You will get a changed reaction, a negative or 'no' response indicating damaged tissue. As you continue to hold the pendulum over your hand you will notice, after a brief interval, the movement beginning to change, gradually returning to the original positive reaction.

To make a complete pendulum diagnosis of a person, you can have your subject lying flat on his back, and then on his face so you can test each part of his body. You may find certain organs are unhealthy, giving a 'no' reaction, and, in particular, areas of the spine where there appear to be problems, possibly due to past strains. The areas you want to test can be located by pointing with the forefinger of your free hand as you ask the question: 'Is the organ to which my finger is pointing healthy?' This same technique may be used if your subject prefers to sit rather than lie down. Actually, some naturopaths do not use the subject himself, employing a 'witness' instead. This 'witness', perhaps a blood sample or a lock of hair, is held in the same hand as the pendulum which is held over an anatomical chart.

Once the unhealthy areas of the body are identified, remedies can be chosen in the ways outlined earlier in this chapter. Perhaps the most common is to have a list of remedies, each one being either pointed at or thought about in turn as the pendulum is held over the affected area. The question being asked is: 'Will this remedy restore this damaged tissue to a healthy state?'

A dental diagnosis and treatment is handled similarly. You may place your forefinger against each tooth in turn. Should a tooth be unsound, the response changes from positive to negative. If the tooth is causing pain, a remedy to relieve the toothache can be identified by mentally running through the list of possibilities. It is quite interesting to do a self-diagnosis of your teeth before you visit the dentist for a check-up. Often, you will be amazed at how accurate your pendulum analysis has been.

HAND AND FOOT CHARTS

A rather different approach to diagnosis involves use of the fingers and different parts of the hand for testing out some of the principle organs of the body. Hand charts such as that illustrated on the next page have been used by dowsers to identify the points on the hands which represent different organs. They suggest these points can be used as 'witnesses'.

Foot charts, too, exist to serve the same purpose, an area which will be more fully explored in the chapter on Reflexology. The problem is that these charts often contradict each other so one feels somewhat dubious about their value. However, one aspect which does seem of value concerns the tip of the big toe or the tip of the thumb. These are seen as representing the 'general polarity' of the body. That is, by dowsing the tip of the thumb or big toe you can get an overall measure of a person's general health, of whether his nervous system is in a correct state of balance. If the reading indicates poor health, a remedy can be chosen by testing it over the person's big toe or thumb.

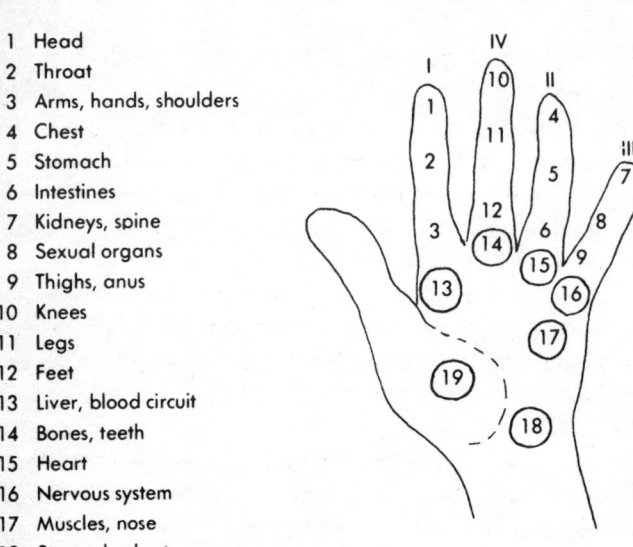

1 Head
2 Throat
3 Arms, hands, shoulders
4 Chest
5 Stomach
6 Intestines
7 Kidneys, spine
8 Sexual organs
9 Thighs, anus
10 Knees
11 Legs
12 Feet
13 Liver, blood circuit
14 Bones, teeth
15 Heart
16 Nervous system
17 Muscles, nose
18 Stomach, chest
19 Throat

If the pendulum gives a positive response over the palm of hand, the patient is in good health. If it doesn't apply the pendulum to each number in turn to locate the defective part. This you identify by the negative response.

Pendulum diagnosis as outlined in this section is interesting and often surprisingly accurate, but is no substitute for examination by a competent doctor. However, as with the dental situation, it is often very useful to do either a self-diagnosis, which is rather limited, or have someone else do a pendulum diagnosis for you. Armed with this information, you can ask your doctor to pay particular attention to areas which have tested negatively. Medical examinations are sometimes very quick and cursory, completely missing indications of potential health troubles. Through use of the pendulum as a check, you can insist on a more thorough examination. If you are proven wrong, no harm has been done. However, if you are right in detecting a trouble spot, you have helped yourself. You have taken a more active role in contributing to your good health and that is what this book is all about.

DOWSING YOUR VITAMINS

When you are interested in testing your body to ascertain its state of health you do have assistance. The medical profession has skills to help you. However, when it comes to the area of vitamins you are unlikely to get any guidance from that direction. Len Thomas found that out quite quickly.

Len felt he needed Vitamin C. Many of the articles he read in various magazines reported studies with this vitamin which applied, so he thought, to his own situation. He bruised easily, had several colds each year and, when he cut himself, often developed an infection in the wound. Len wanted to use Vitamin C in an attempt to combat these problems but was uncertain about dosage. How could he determine the optimum amount to take?

First of all he asked his doctor. He got no help there, for the doctor told him vitamins were a waste of time and money, suggesting that Len simply take prescribed medication whenever he developed an infection or bad bruising. Being a persistent fellow, Len did not accept this view because he was interested in preventing his problems rather than treating them after they appeared. He asked the proprietor of his local health food store, but this advice was rather confusing, leaving Len still uncertain over the potency of tablet he should take and the dosage. Also, he had a vague feeling that the proprietor was more interested in potential profit than in Len's health. Suggestions provided by magazine articles added to the confusion, because they seemed to contradict each other. Similarly, advice from friends, though well-meaning, did not help greatly because of their lack of knowledge.

Len was confused. He was intelligent enough to realize that what is a tolerable amount of a substance for one person might be detrimental for someone else, and that a person's requirements could change from time to time. This point seems to be sometimes overlooked when drugs are prescribed, the assumption being that the drug works the same for everyone irrespective of personal variables. This is one explanation of side effects which can be damaging to one person but not another. With vitamins the problem is not so criticial, for their capacity for doing harm is minimal. In practice, it is obvious that we can vary greatly in our needs and our ability to utilize the substances we take into our bodies be they food, drugs or vitamin pills. The great number of people affected, even hospitalized, as a direct result of prescribed medications attests to the amount of guesswork in medical practice. Yet, of course, such guesses may be the best anyone could give because we just do not know what a specific person should take and in what quantity he should take it.

By chance, Len's wife told him how a friend of hers used a pendulum to decide on her daily vitamin intake. She thought it was a great joke but Len was interested. After finding out more about it from his wife's friend, he saw dowsing as a possible means of learning about his body's needs. It was clear to him that many people were on a steady diet of vitamin and mineral supplements in the mistaken belief that they were necessary, without any idea whether they were proving of value or not. Conversely, other people either took no such supplements, or in amounts too small to be of any benefit. Measuring by means of the pendulum would make it possible to establish, Len realized, whether in the body there existed a need, a balance, or a surplus of any particular substance.

USING CHARTS AS AN AID TO DIAGNOSIS

Some people find that using a chart such as the one on the page opposite, which was provided by Finch in *The Pendulum and Your Health* helps them to establish their body's condition.

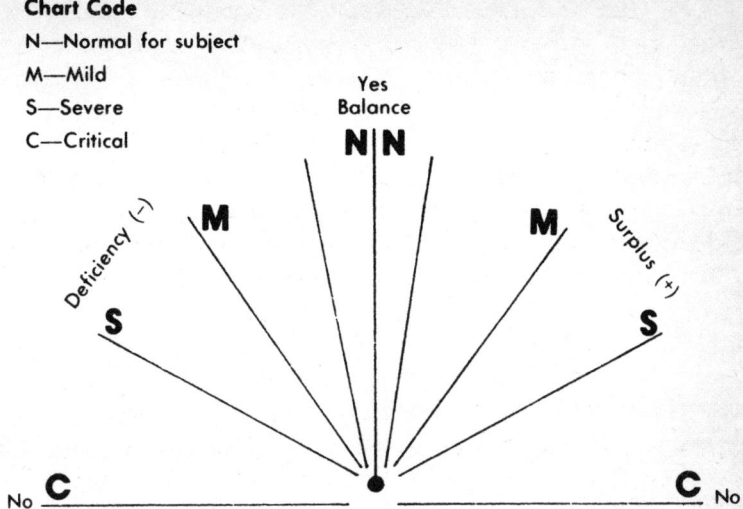

The pendulum is suspended over the starting point, and, as in Len's case, the question would be asked: 'Do I have an ideal balance of Vitamin C in my body?'. According to Finch's chart, the pendulum would swing vertically if the answer was 'yes'. Should Len's body lack Vitamin C, the pendulum would swing into the left hand side of the chart, indicating the degree of deficiency as mild, severe, or critical. If Len had a surplus of Vitamin C, the pendulum would swing into the right hand side of the chart. Further questioning would determine the amount of the vitamin necessary to restore the balance.

Charts can be quite elaborate but, personally, I do not find them very helpful. In Len's situation, I would be inclined to ask: 'Does my body require Vitamin C at this moment?'. If the response was 'yes', I would ask whether my body required half a gram, three-quarters of a gram, a gram and so on until I ascertained the amount the pendulum considered I needed. You can use the actual bottle of vitamin pills when asking your questions, but it is easier to make up a list of supplements you might possibly need and ask about each one individually.

Further, you can find whether it is preferable to take a particular tablet with, before, or after meals, or whether it should be taken in the morning, noon or evening. Charts are not needed to gain such information in my opinion but, again, *you* might enjoy using them.

One thing to watch, though, is that you should set up your charts to conform to your pendulum responses. On Finch's chart, the negative response is from side-to-side and the positive response is to-and-fro. This is the opposite of my own pendulum reactions, and would create a source of confusion.

TWO FINAL IDEAS

An idea you might care to investigate. Our digestive systems are made up of two separate operations. We have an acid process in which the enzymes in our bodies digest protein, and an alkaline process which acts upon the carbohydrates. These systems should be in balance if good health is to be maintained, though normally we have no way of ascertaining this. Accordingly, you can use your pendulum to determine your acid/alkaline balance by asking questions such as: 'Is my acid/alkaline balance correct? Too acid? Too alkaline?'

To remedy the situation, you can run through a list of foods asking what you should eat to restore the balance. If you wish, you can even set up a body acidity scale, say with 100 as a mid-point. Below 100 represents alkalinity and above 100 represents acidity. Starting at 50, you could enquire whether your acidity level was 50, 60, 70 etc. until you received a positive response. This would indicate the extent of imbalance in your body.

A final point concerns weight control plans. You might like to set up 100% as a point of total success. You could then test out a diet plan before you embarked upon it, asking 'Will this plan be 100% successful in achieving my desired weight? 90%? 80%?' and so on. Several possible plans could be checked in this way and the one with the likelihood of highest success selected. Similarly, the pendulum could be used to check your choice of food items within a diet, providing an answer to the question: 'Is it in my best interest to eat . .?

Pendulum dowsing, then, can be and has been used in a variety of ways to help people improve their health. It provides information which may be unavailable in other ways. You may feel it is ridiculous to use such a method to prescribe for yourself. Well and good, do not bother about it. Perhaps ideas you come across in other chapters will be more acceptable. Perhaps you feel sceptical but are prepared to give it a trial. Do so by all means and you may find you are surprised by the results. Maybe you're full of enthusiasm. Great, but do not get too carried away. Pendulum dowsing is fallible. You'll make mistakes. We all do. Use it sensibly, trying to check the results you get in other ways. Certainly, it would be unwise to depend upon it solely in cases of serious health problems where medical advice is available. It is a tool which, if used intelligently, may well guide you towards improved health in the day-to-day choices you are called upon to make. In addition, you will probably enjoy yourself learning a new skill. The next chapter, too, presents a new skill in which you might be interested, that of acupressure and reflex therapy.

8. Healing through Finger Pressure

PRESSURE POINT THERAPY

Acupressure, or pressure point therapy, is a do-it-yourself treatment method which involves pressing your finger tips upon certain contact points in the body which are said to relate to various glands and organs. If the particular body area, gland or organ is malfunctioning in some way, the contact point representing it will be painful, sensitive to the touch. This soreness is seen as indicating an energy leak which must be rectified if the malfunction is to be corrected. This is done by exerting firm pressure with the finger tip to close the leak, allowing energy to flow back into the part of the body which was losing it. Often, a feeling of warmth accompanies the treatment, this being taken as a sign that healing is taking place. Once the tenderness has disappeared from any spot being treated, it is assumed regeneration is complete. This usually occurs after a number of finger pressure sessions, single treatment cures being rather rare.

In his book, *The Natural Healers Acupressure Handbook*, Michael Blate explains the rationale behind this treatment method in terms of life energy. He suggests that the nature of our health is a reflection of the state of the bioenergy which surrounds us. We are, according to this theory, living in a 'sea of energy' which constantly permeates our bodies. This universal essence of life is seen as following a predictable route through our bodies, flowing along a pathway which follows a fixed pattern. There are twelve major organs and organ functions in the body where the bioenergy appears to change direction, the pathway dividing into major routes called meridians. Along these meridians exist numerous interconnections called acupoints.

Although the nature of bioenergy is to flow smoothly and harmoniously through the body, it may be disturbed due to the body's inner environment becoming out of balance with its external environment. The acupoints along the circuit act to correct the disturbed energy flow, but if this rebalancing is not effected quickly, organ malfunction is likely to occur resulting in ill-health and disease.

In terms of this theory, curing a disease requires correction of the imbalance between internal and external environments which is the cause of the problem. Often a change in lifestyle may be necessary to restore harmony. More specific treatment may centre on the acupoints, for their role in determining how bioenergy reaches the organs is vital. Manipulative techniques may be used to stimulate these points, possibly the best known being acupuncture in which needles are the instruments employed. However, heat, sound, ice, electricity and fingertips may also be used to manipulate the acupoints in an effort to restore harmony to the body system.

Acupressure, which has been described as fingertip acupuncture, is a harmless first-aid treatment which is intended primarily for basically healthy people. That is, it is not a recommended approach for chronic, long-standing problems. Nor should it be used if you have a heart condition, chronic arthritis or cancer. Should you be on a regime of daily medication, acupressure is unsuited to you, for it is not recommended for use within four hours of taking any drugs, medications or intoxicants. Nor is it a suggested treatment for women after the third month of pregnancy, or if the indicated pressure point lies upon the breast. In fact, pressure points lying beneath scars, warts, moles, varicose veins or inflamed skin are best avoided. Blate suggests, too, that should your emotional state be very agitated, you would be well-advised to postpone acupressure treatment until you feel more tranquil.

If it be thought that too many people are thus precluded from using this approach to health improvement, it is well to remember that most of the problems which plague us are relatively minor disturbances of an otherwise healthy state. Acupressure has a wide range of applicability, particularly since many of the points act to remove a range of symptoms. In this respect, they are somewhat comparable to the homoeopathic polycrests described on page 61.

Ideally, if pressure point stimulation is effective, immediate symptom relief is gained on the first treatment. This is followed by further gradual easing of discomfort. Often, though certainly not always, the entire body feels more relaxed, much tension seeming to drain away. It is rare for the symptom to disappear entirely after the initial pressure treatment. However, when it does return, it is less severe. The same point which provided initial relief should again be stimulated. This procedure is followed on three or four occasions by which time the symptom has probably disappeared. If it has not done so, and persists in recurring, it is wise to see your doctor. Acupressure therapy, like all other methods described in this book, is a first step measure, to be used before more powerful agents such as drugs are employed. If these natural, harmless treatments do not effect the desired healing, orthodox medicine is indicated as the next step.

IMPORTANT ACUPRESSURE POINTS

For the layman, the greatest problem with this therapy method is the great number of points involved. These can run into the hundreds, depending on the particular book you read. The average person would, I feel, give up in dismay when faced by the myriad diagrams purporting to show him how to find the fifteen points necessary to stimulate for, say, headache relief. Therefore, I have attempted to abstract some of the more important acupressure points, ones which have a wide range of action and which are relatively easy to locate. Should you, as a result of trying out this system of healing, wish to extend your knowledge by learning the location and action of more points, I suggest you read Blate's book which is both comprehensive and easy to follow. Although he provides detailed information on many acupressure points, there are six which he stresses because of their general usefulness.

The first of these is located two thumb widths above the most prominent crease of the outer wrist, in line with the middle finger.

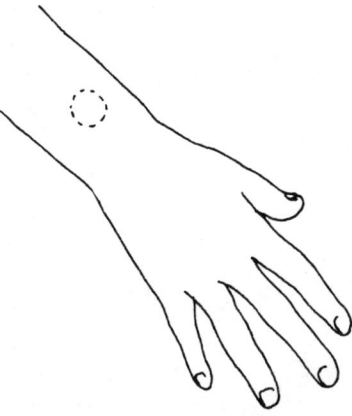

This point is particularly valuable for problems of the chest, shoulder, arm, elbow and wrist. It is also likely to provide relief from facial neuralgia, headaches and ear problems, as well as from cold symptoms. Coughs and sore throats, for example, have been relieved through pressure on this point.

A second important location is in the hollow behind the crown of the outer ankle.

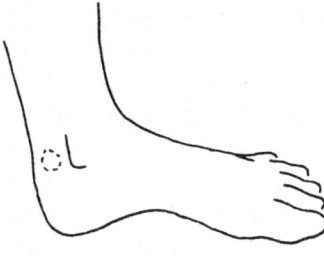

Leg problems, particularly muscular spasms and strains, often yield to pressure upon this point. Other ailments likely to respond are painful lower backs, haemorrhoids, eczema, headache, neuralgia and toothache.

Another point which is of use in a wide variety of ailments is found at the width of one hand above the crown of the inner ankle, just behind the shin bone.

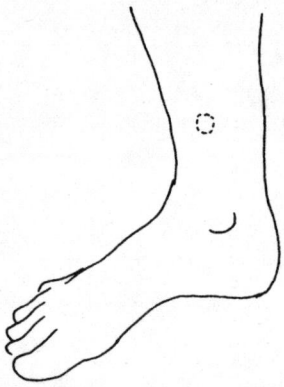

Stimulation of this point is often combined with that of the one to be described next to cope with abdominal and stomach disorders such as diarrhoea, flatulence, indigestion and vomiting. Lower back discomfort and hip pain also may yield to stimulation of these two points. Treated alone, this point has produced marked benefit in relieving nausea of various types, including that of travel sickness, as well as helping in the relief of constipation, leg and foot problems and the pain associated with menstruation.

Point number four is found the width of one hand below the bottom of the kneecap; then one thumb's width towards the outside of the leg. It lies in the valley beside the shin bone and, as well as its already commented upon value in abdominal and stomach disorders, often provides an effective treatment for back, hip, leg and foot problems. The symptoms of colds, influenza, coughs, fatigue, heat rash and headache may be treated by pressure on this point, and, like the one previously described, it has been successfully used for the relief of travel sickness.

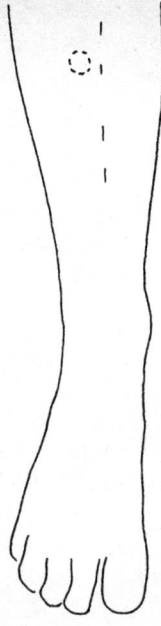

Found the width of two thumbs above the most prominent crease on the inner wrist, in line with the middle finger, this next point has a wide variety of applications ranging from abdominal pains, diarrhoea, vomiting and retching, travel sickness, arm and hand problems (especially swollen armpit) through coughs, chest and respiratory complaints, heartburn, to insomnia and menstruation problems.

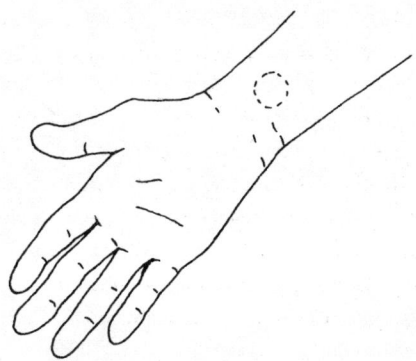

The final key point is located on the hand in the webbing between the thumb and forefinger which should be squeezed together. Your finger is then placed on top of the mound so formed. As the hand is relaxed your fingers should remain on the correct place to stimulate.

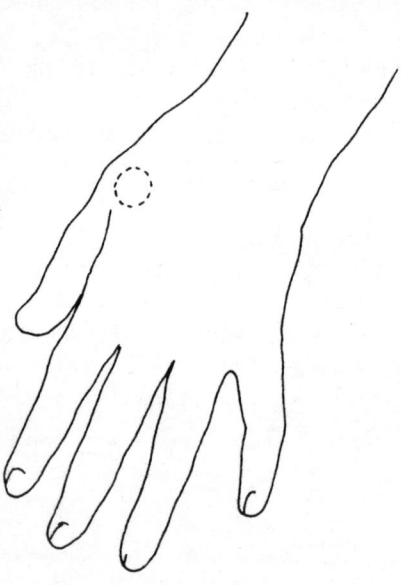

This acupressure point is used primarily for complaints from the chest upwards, so the mouth, face and head are all included in its action. Respiratory problems, sinusitis, and catarrh, colds, influenza, ear and eye troubles, sore throat, laryngitis, migraine, neck tension, heat rash, facial neuralgia and headache may all find relief through pressure on this point.

It will have become obvious, even from this very brief description, that the same ailments recur with each point. That is because these six points are central to the practice of acupressure therapy and their range of application is so broad. The appropriate procedure to follow is try one point and await results. If it has not produced the relief you seek, try the next. Stimulation of one or another is likely to contribute to the removal of your symptom.

Points should be stimulated bilaterally. Most acupressure

points, with the exception of those lying along the spine or the front mid line of the body, are duplicated on either side of the body, on both legs, both arms, or both hands. It is important to treat both points, using fingertips, thumb or knuckle. Hold your finger vertical and move it in a circle. Blate suggests an anti-clockwise direction but others recommend clockwise, so you can make your own choice.

Press hard. People are usually too gentle and often do little more than rub the fingertip over the skin. Skin and fingertip should move together as you keep the pressure on for 15 to 20 seconds. Move then to the bilateral point and stimulate for the same amount of time. Relax and wait until some relief is felt. When this occurs, begin gently to use the injured area until full movement is restored.

Although the diagrams given to help you locate the acupressure points will be useful, your body is your best guide. As you deeply probe around the area indicated in the diagrams, you will feel a tenderness, a sensitivity. This is the exact point to stimulate, even if it does not seem to exactly match the illustration. If your treatment is successful, this soreness will either disappear, or become less intense.

REFLEX THERAPY

It may seem difficult to accept that stimulation of a point on your hand will exert a healing influence on, say, your teeth. Yet validity of this principle has been demonstrated repeatedly.

Kerry Abbott's face ached. Normally she took aspirin under such circumstances but one of the girls with whom she played tennis told her about acupressure therapy. Kerry thought it was worth a try for she would be no worse off if it failed. She could always use aspirin, although she was becoming increasingly uneasy about the number of these to which she resorted whenever pain occurred. Rather sceptically she tried the first of the points described, stimulating it on both arms. Her scepticism was confirmed. No pain relief resulted. However, treatment of the point described on page 127 produced an effect. The pain did not disappear entirely, but it became bearable. In fact it continued to deminish and a further treatment an hour later continued this process.

Since the time of her introduction to acupressure treatment, Kerry has become very interested in the reflex principle of healing. She found that, should one of her sons be troubled by a foreign body in an eye, rubbing the other eye acted reflexively, causing tears to flow which washed away the irritant. Her husband's painful right hip, legacy of an old football injury, often responded favourably to treatment of tender spots in his right shoulder. These tender spots sometimes disappeared after finger manipulation. On other occasions, pressure on the joints of the small toes where they joined the foot, or on the joints of the little fingers where they joined the hand proved more effective.

Hot water may serve as an alternative to finger pressure. Kerry's husband discovered, virtually by accident, that the best treatment for the pain he experienced in his right shoulder was to keep dipping his right hand and wrist into very hot water. The water was not sufficiently hot to cause scalding but was as hot as he could bear. Similarly, when any member of Kerry's family had toothache, she would apply hot fomentations to the side of the face opposite from that where the trouble was. This usually relieved pain more effectively than applying them to the site of the actual toothache itself. If the sufferer also took hot foot baths, pain relief was speeded up. It has been well known for centuries that treating the feet in this way affects the head, relieving complaints localized in this part of the body. Headaches, ear problems, head colds, nasal congestion, and a myriad of other ailments seem to improve through treatment with hot foot baths. When the problem is sinusitis, pressure exerted just behind the angle of the jaw, in the hollows behind each ear, has often proven beneficial.

Conversely, ice may also be used as a supplement to finger pressure. After one 15–20 second treatment with the finger or thumb, apply an ice cube to the acupressure point. Keep it moving in small circles as you press it on the point for approximately 30 seconds. Then, warm the area within your hand before repeating the procedure. Ice packs to the base of

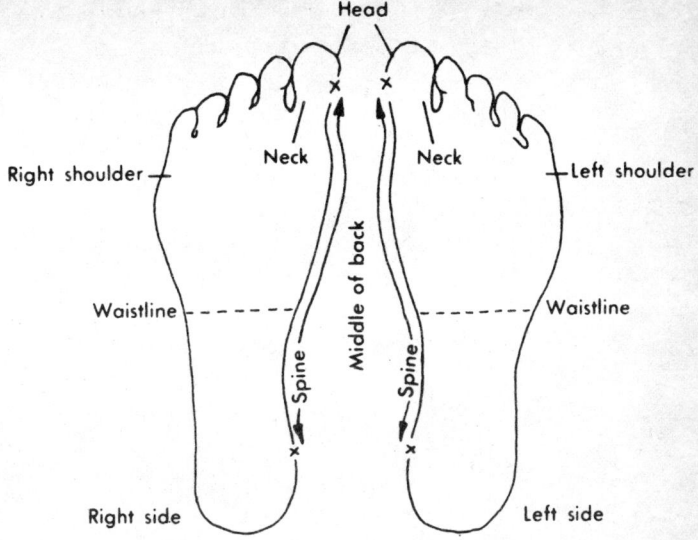

the skull, another ancient remedy, can work reflexively, benefiting the whole body, releasing tension and helping to overcome fatigue.

Fingertips, thumbs, hot water and ice are only some of the 'tools' used to practise reflex therapy which might generally be defined as seeking to relieve or eliminate symptoms through stimulating parts of the body different from that where the symptom is physically located. Knuckles, golf balls, aluminium combs, elastic bands and clothes pegs are all used to exert pressure on acupoints. Practitioners of 'zone therapy' make frequent use of such 'instruments'.

ZONE THERAPY

This term, derived from the work of Dr William Fitzgerald earlier this century, systematizes the pressure relationships so far discussed in this chapter. Fitzgerald's theory divides the human body longitudinally into five zones on the left and five on the right. Individual zones may be traced from each finger and corresponding toe, passing through the various organs located therein.

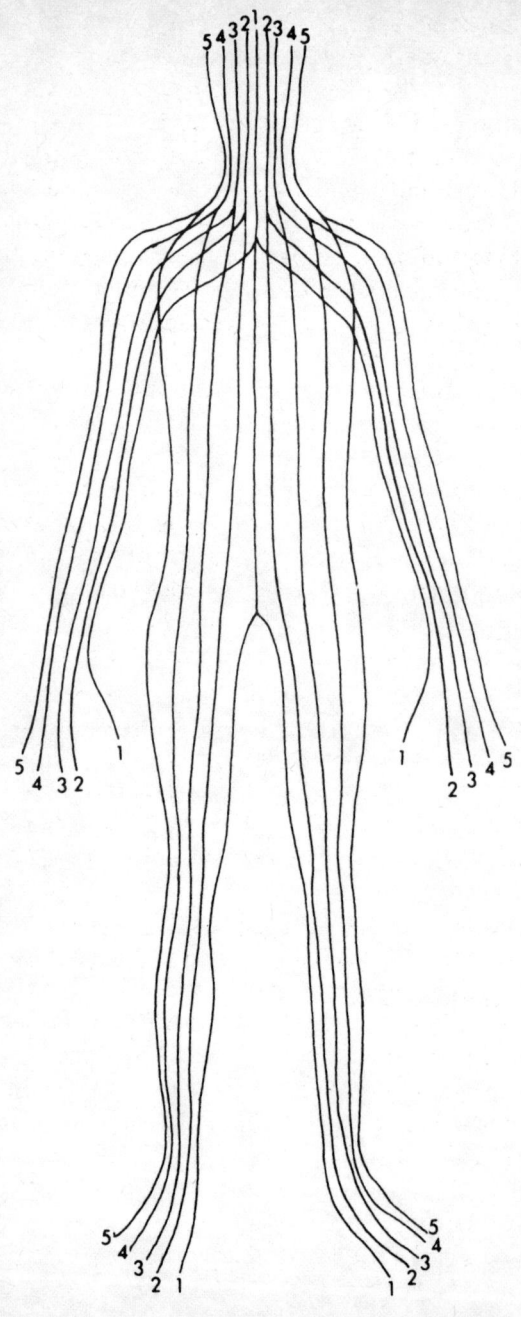

Thus, the zone from the little finger and small toe passes up and down the outside of the body, affecting the shoulder, ear, hip and skin. The zone from the thumb and big toe passes through the bladder and stomach while those from the third and fourth right fingers and toes passes through the liver and right kidney. Similarly those from the left hand pass through the left kidney, heart and spleen. Pressure on any point in one of these longitudinal zones is theorized as affecting all organs in the same zone by reflex action. Therefore, a problem occurring anywhere within a zone may be treated by pressure somewhere else within that zone.

No one really knows why this type of therapy works. Zones, meridians and reflex action have not really been convincingly explained, and in this respect, are akin to many other treatments outlined in this book. Again, we are faced with the recurrent situation of a thing working without anyone really knowing why it works. Why, for example, should pressure applied to the second toe of the left foot help relieve a stomach ache? Why should pressure just below the big toe exert an effect on the spinal column at shoulder level? Yet, the system seems to work, and has done for so many years. To find whether it will do so for you is an activity involving no risk to yourself. The method is harmless and only benefit can result. Even if you miss the precise pressure point, the body's reflexes seem to operate in such a way that your manipulation is likely to produce a good result. If it does not, you will not be inflicting any damage.

Zone therapy emphasizes the importance of the hands and feet, for these are parts of the body where nerves and nerve endings are close to the skin surface. Thus, they are more accessible to manipulation and massage. Although the same reflexes are present in both hands and feet, they are more difficult to locate in the former than the latter. Because we work with our hands, the reflexes are not as sensitive as they are in the feet. Shoes keep our feet in a tender condition, so it is relatively easy to locate areas which require treatment.

The feet, according to 'zone therapy' theory, are reflections of all the organs in the body, as are the hands. Precise 'maps' of

132 The Healing Factor

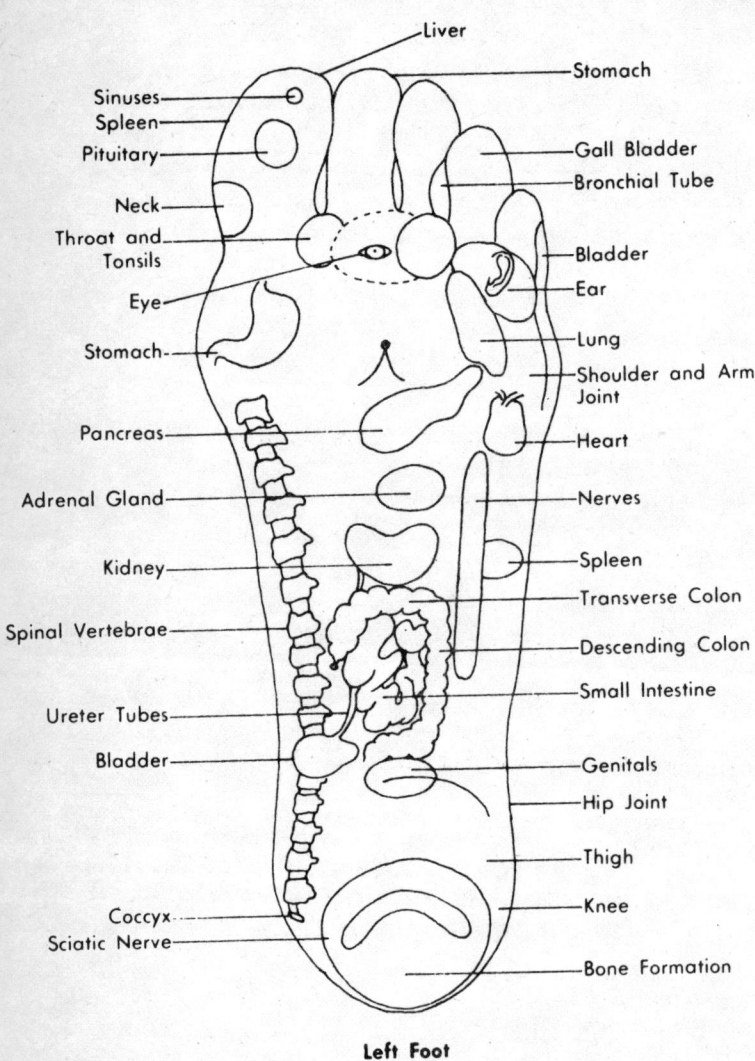

Left Foot

(After Brodsky. *From Eden to Aquarius*, pp. 221-222.)

Healing Through Finger Pressure 133

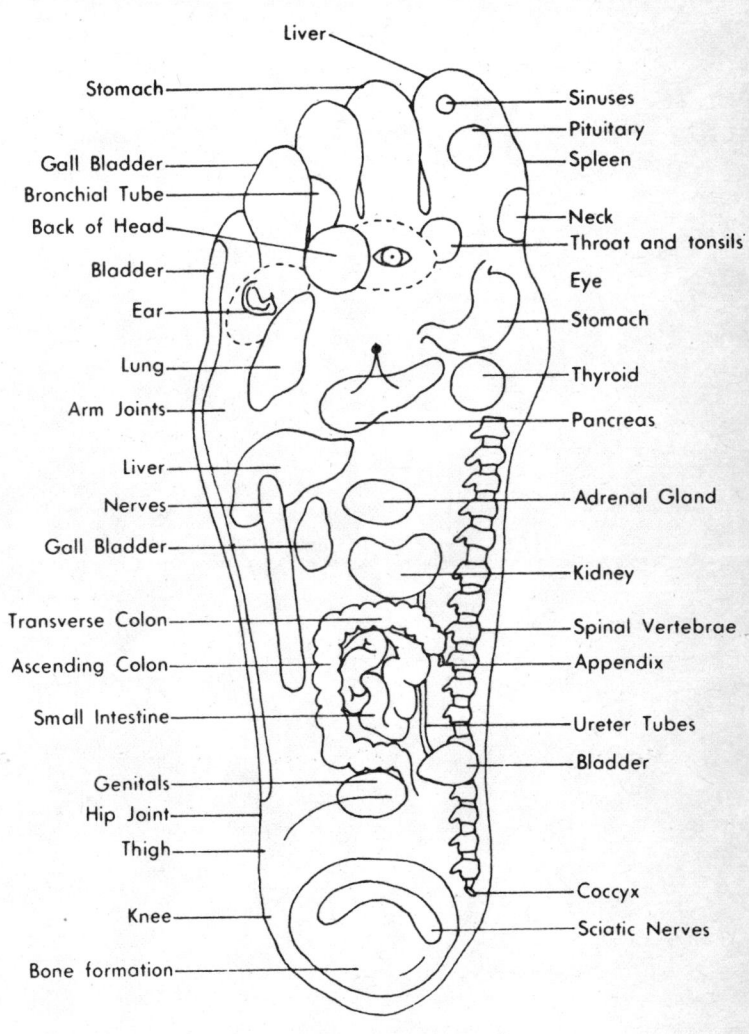

Right Foot

134 The Healing Factor

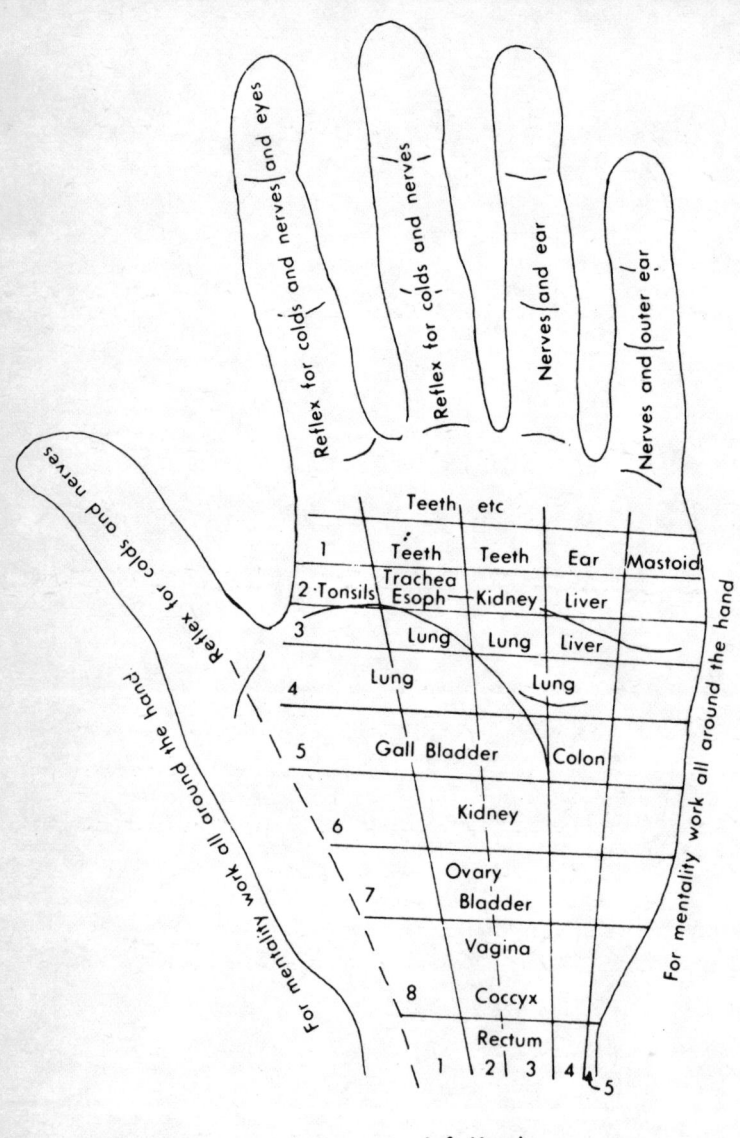

Left Hand

Comparable locations are found upon the hands.

Healing Through Finger Pressure

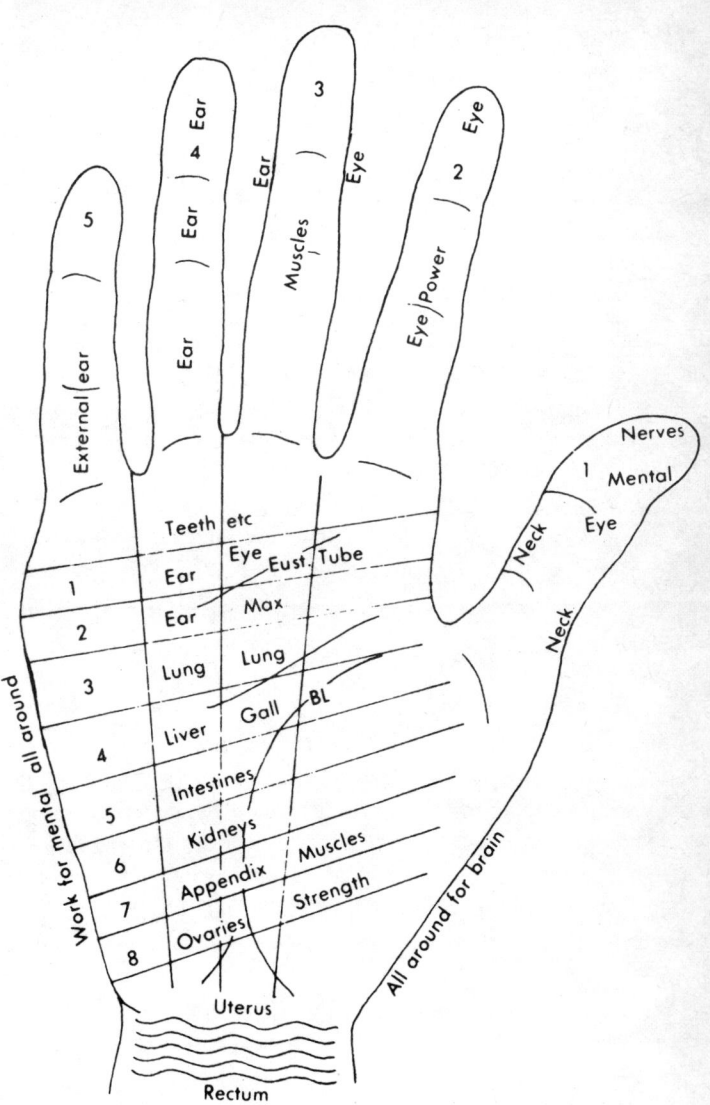

Right Hand

the soles of the feet are available, showing the areas which should be stimulated in order to promote healing of particular parts of the body. As each foot is divided into five zones, and as treatment of any area within a zone produces an effect on every part of the body within that zone, it does provide a convenient area upon which pressure may be exerted. The problem is that the 'maps' vary somewhat, with particular body organs appearing in different locations. Such disagreements are, however, minor and there is general consensus upon basic locations. These are given in the diagrams on pages 132 and 133..

The appropriate zones may also be reached from the top of the foot, the areas to be treated lying directly above the corresponding area on the sole of the foot. Actually, precision in the 'mapping' of the organs is not critical for, as with the acupressure therapy outlined earlier, the body provides its own location information. By applying pressure with the thumb, which is usually the best 'instrument' when treating the feet, sensitive spots give the 'ouch' response. If areas respond with soreness when probed with minimal pressure, this would suggest your health is capable of considerable improvement. Stimulating these tender areas could well be the means of achieving this.

Though the thumb usually provides the best treatment, alternatives are available. The rubber eraser on the end of a pencil might be used to exert more pressure for deeper massage, and, if the hands rather than the feet are being treated, rubber bands can be employed to provide a constant pressure. They are wound around the joints of specific fingers. Another way of maintaining a strong, steady pressure on the fingers is through the use of clothespegs which are applied primarily to the tips. When pressure is to be exerted on the hand over a wide area, an aluminium comb works very well. This is held in the palm and the fingers closed around its teeth. These are all very simple techniques. In fact, perhaps the chief virtue of zone therapy is its simplicity, for anyone can begin self-treatment so easily, the rewards being quite out of proportion to the little effort required.

When treating a particular area, it is necessary to cover all the zones in which an organ may lie. The liver, for example, spreads across all five zones on the right hand side of the body and zones one and two on the left hand side. All these should be massaged on the sole of the foot. In cases where internal organs are being treated, front and back zones are massaged simultaneously. Pain existing anywhere in zone one, for example, can usually be relieved by pressure exerted on the big toe. If this pressure is applied to the underside of the toe, only the back of the body in zone one will be affected. It is necessary to treat the top and tip of the big toe as well to ensure complete coverage of the zone.

In fact, probably the most effective way of using the zone therapy principle is to massage the soles of the feet, and the top of the feet, too, for about ten minutes each day. If possible, take a hot foot bath to relax the tissues before you begin. Tender spots identified during the treatment should receive special attention for they draw attention to ailing parts of the body. Massage is usually best done with the thumbs but an alternative is to roll a golf ball back and forth under the feet. This can be done while watching television and the technique ensures that quite deep pressure is exerted all over the foot. Walking barefooted along beaches will accomplish the same result whereby all the body's zones receive stimulation.

When treating organs and parts of the body which are in pairs, such as lungs, kidneys, shoulders, eyes, treat the appropriate areas in both feet even when it is only one side of the body which is ailing. This applies also to single organs such as the thyroid gland and the stomach which have locations 'mapped' in both feet.

Probe the soles of the feet deeply, applying pressure where pain is greatest. Even if you are in some doubt about what the painful spot indicates, what organ malfunction it reflects, you can go ahead and massage the area. The sensitivity suggests that something is wrong and a series of treatments to reduce and remove the pain can only prove beneficial.

SOME SPECIFIC APPLICATIONS OF ZONE THERAPY

I know of several families who adopt the experimental approach. If any member of the family has an ailment, the appropriate reflex on the sole of the foot is massaged by another family member. Results are then awaited. Should no improvement be apparent, the hand reflex is tried. If this, too, is ineffective, the acupressure points are treated. It is a surprisingly rare occurrence for this approach to meet with failure.

One such family, that of Hans and Marlene Brandt, have been practitioners for the best part of thirty years. Like many other healing practices, acupressure and zone therapy have enjoyed wide acceptance in Europe, and the Brandts carried their beliefs with them when they immigrated to Australia. So effective have they been in relieving the common ailments of their friends and neighbours that, at least in their suburb, acupressure and zone therapy have become a basic first step treatment. Should it prove ineffective in a particular case, then orthodox medical help is sought.

Excessive nervousness, tension and anxiety, problems so often mentioned in these pages, have little place in the Brandt household. Their routine ten-minute foot massage each evening is probably the main reason, but should a stressful situation arise in the life of any family member, rubber bands are placed on the first, second and third fingers of both hands. These remain in place for up to fifteen minutes. An alternative treatment for nervousness is to place clothespegs on the finger and thumb tips, again for approximately fifteen minutes. Should discomfort be felt, remove the rubber bands and clothes pegs more quickly, but treat yourself to several short sessions instead of the longer one. Even interlocking the fingers and exerting pressure by squeezing as hard as possible for several minutes at a time may improve your ability to handle the stress problem. Should fatigue be associated with your tension, use a hair comb to stroke the palm of your hand upwards from fingertips to wrist for a minute or two.

Back problems, so common in our society, are rarely found in the Brandt family circle. Hans, whose work as a storeman, involves a lot of heavy lifting, occasionally suffers minor strains but he uses the spinal reflex to treat these. As the spinal column is located in the exact centre of the body, the reflex for it lies along the first zone of each foot. The big toe represents the head and the centre of the foot is the centre of the back. This provides a guide for Hans to locate the precise spot on his foot to manipulate to relieve his back pain. Should his pain be more general, less easy to pinpoint, he follows the spinal reflex down towards his heel until he probes a tender spot. This he massages very gently. As the tenderness lessens, he applies more pressure.

Hans can do no damage by over massaging this reflex. That is true for most other reflexes also, although the liver and kidney should be treated with care. Brief massage only is indicated for these two reflexes as overstimulation can, on occasions, lead to a nauseous feeling.

Though the Brandt's children do suffer from the normal colds, coughs and sore throats, they seem to recover from these more quickly than their schoolmates. At the first sign of a cold, Marlene massages their toes and, briefly, the lung and kidney reflexes. Should the throat be painful, she concentrates upon the throat reflex in the fleshy part of the big toe. Since the discomfort usually lies in the front part of the throat, the pressure is exerted on the top of the toe just where it meets the foot. Massaging this area between thumb and forefinger is often very effective.

Should sinusitis be the problem, the big toe again comes in for special attention, although any toe which reveals tenderness is massaged. Pressing the area at the base of the big toe and that between the second and third toes often helps in the relief of sinus discomfort. Hayfever can be relieved in this way, too, as it can by pressure applied to the thumbs and first fingers with clothespegs.

One of the Brandt's neighbours, who was becoming increasingly hard of hearing, tried zone therapy as a possible avenue of improvement. He pressed the teeth of an aluminium comb against his finger tips for a period of five minutes at a time. In addition he squeezed the joints of his third (ring) fingers and third toes. He felt he gained some benefit from this treatment, certainly more than from anything else he had tried.

Ear problems generally show up as tenderness between the fourth and fifth toes. Massage of this area until the tenderness disappears is likely to bring relief, as is five minutes use of a clothespeg on the tip of the third fingers. The waists of the three middle toes, too, are ear reflexes, and manipulation of these often produces positive results.

This is true for eye complaints, also, although the main area of treatment would be the bottom of these toes. It is helpful to massage this area using two fingers in a rolling motion, pressing down hard to find and eliminate the sore spot. The corresponding area on the top of the foot could beneficially be included in this manipulation. For eye strain, tight squeezing of the knuckles of the first fingers of both hands has been known to effect improvement. Pressure on the joints of the first and second fingers could be valuable if you have sties, granulated lids or conjunctivitis. Alternatively, try an elastic band wrapped firmly around the thumb at the base of the nail for about five minutes.

There are many other complaints which may be treated through zone therapy. Nervous or spasmodic conditions such as hiccoughs are usually relieved by a few minutes pressure and deep massage on the centre of the soles of the feet. Headaches often respond well to massage of the big toe. The pain of haemorrhoids may yield to pressure exerted down towards the heel. Use your thumb and index finger, working your way around the heels of both feet and press in firmly towards the bone.

If you have an infection, you can massage the lymph gland and kidney reflexes. Proceed slowly here, perhaps only a minute or so for the first couple of days until the tenderness becomes less noticeable. Leg cramps, or cramps anywhere in the body, may be treated by clasping and squeezing the Achilles tendon, while vague back and neck pains are often relieved by using your knuckles to press strongly against the sole of your foot. In addition, use the knuckles of your other hand to loosen the ligaments of the top of the foot directly above the area you are working on.

There are myriad other applications of the reflex principle. *Zone Therapy*, written by Bergon and Tuchack, provides a comprehensive list of common ailments, devoting a short chapter to the treatment of each of these. This book would be of interest if you wish to pursue further this approach to self-healing. Their suggestions are easy to follow. One of the main virtues of acupressure and reflex therapy is that it is so simple. Also, you find out very quickly whether the method is helpful to you or not. Some people, such as the Brandt's, see it as the best natural treatment system there is. Others try it, and find it does not produce the expected results. Some are disappointed when they treat themselves, but then find good results coming when another person massages their feet. Try it both ways, as a self-help treatment and as a family-helping-each-other programme. Possibly you will find zone therapy works well for some ailments and not for others. Test it out and, as with all the other approaches described in this book, use that which produces positive results for *you*.

Part 3
Developing a Healthy Lifestyle

9. Nutritional Health

THE IMPORTANCE OF NUTRITION

Many of us worry about our weight, so we tend to know something about diet, which may be defined as our daily intake of food and drink. Nutrition is a broader concept, embracing all the processes involved in using foodstuffs for the body's growth, maintenance and repair. As such, it is of vast importance to our health, yet we do not know very much about it.

Unfortunately, the average general medical practitioner will be able to add little to our inadequate store of knowledge. Most doctors are in no position to offer advice on the food which is best for you to eat, for medical schools have traditionally ignored the subject of nutrition. The physicians they train, naturally, regard it of little importance, probably knowing less about it than the waiter or waitress who serves you in a restaurant. A study conducted at Harvard by Dr Jean Mayer, Professor of Nutrition at that university, found that the average doctor knows a little more about nutrition than his secretary. However, should his secretary have a weight problem, she is likely to know a little more about nutrition than her doctor.

Dr Mayer is on record as saying that: 'The main diseases we deal with and the main causes of death are influenced by nutrition—and they are more easily prevented than treated.' As our medical advisers cannot guide us in the prevention of illness through sound nutritional practices, we need to take responsibility for our own eating habits, and to try and improve upon them.

This is, of course, easy to say but less easy to accomplish. We do become creatures of habit, and find change difficult. It is understandable why doctors prefer to treat an illness once it has developed rather than attempting to prevent that illness. Through antibiotics, for example, they often achieve spectacular instant successes, a circumstance far more gratifying to the ego than the extremely difficult task of trying to change the eating habits of their patients. If they have little success in encouraging people to stop smoking and drinking excessive amounts of alcohol, the results of which practices clearly result in poorer health, what hope have they in attempting to influence people to eat less sugar, salt, and white flour products, when it is far less clear that such a change will result in improved health.

That is indeed a problem in the field of nutrition. There is so much confusion about which foods are good for you and which foods are bad. Experts state their theories with complete assurance as if they were proven facts, quite unperturbed that other experts counsel the opposite. Today, low protein, high carbohydrate diets are becoming increasingly popular; five years ago, high protein, low carbohydrate diets were all the rage. Butter was a villain not so long ago while margarine was a hero. Now it seems the roles are being reversed and by the time this book is published the situation may have changed again. Where are we to turn for guidance if we want to take more responsibility for our health by a more careful selection of the food we eat?

In a previous chapter I talked about using the pendulum to select foods which are in harmony with us. That may help. In this chapter I shall try to guide you through the morass of conflicting claims about the nutritional value of different foods, attempting to identify those about which there is general agreement. There does seem to be considerable agreement about the 'don'ts', the food you should not eat if you wish to prevent illness. Less agreement exists on the 'do's', those foods which actively promote good health, but some useful statements can still be made about them.

If one thing does emerge clearly from a study of nutrition it is that people are becoming increasingly disenchanted with food which is artificially coloured, flavoured and tenderized. An experiment said to illustrate the reason for such disenchantment has been oft reported, but I have been unable to locate the original description. Still it's an amusing story. It involves two groups of chickens. One was fed on a well-known breakfast cereal while the second was fed the shredded empty packet in which the cereal was packaged. The chickens given the cardboard apparently fared better than the ones given the cereal.

Perhaps that is just a tall story, but another example, indicating our attitude to the prevention-treatment issue, is not. A United Nations survey found that tooth decay was much worse in England than in Ghana, except for the wealthier Ghanaians. Their teeth were as cavity-prone as were those of the average Englishman. This wealthy group imported food from England, primarily the sugary, refined foods we love so well. The United Nations' report pointed out these circumstances, expressing concern that as more and more Ghanaians adopted a Western diet, tooth decay would increase dramatically. Their solution? Institute a crash course to train more dentists to deal with the problem once it developed. There was no suggestion that it would be far more effective to prevent the problem developing by curtailing the import of the damaging foods.

So the responsiblity is yours. Nutrition is possibly the field which offers the best opportunity for you to improve your own health through practicing self-help preventive medicine. It has been estimated that you have more than one thousand opportunities a year to do so, based on a three meal a day regime which goes on seven days a week for fifty two weeks of the year. So let us now look at the principles which might provide a guide to you in your self-improvement programme.

THE PRINCIPLES OF GOOD NUTRITION

Jocelyn Gradon is a person who cares about the food she eats. Some might call her a 'crank' or a 'food fadist'. There is a difference, however, in being discriminating about food, about wanting to know what nutriments it contains and which chemicals have been added, and going to unrealistic extremes. It is easy to go too far, adopting a diet which appeals intellectually but which does not suit the body. Jocelyn was not like that. She tried various foods and noted their effect upon her, always listening to her body's messages. Her idea was to find the diet, the particular blend of foods, which helped her feel vibrantly healthy. No one else could do this for her, just as no one else can do it for you.

So, the first principle, once again, is to *be your own expert*. Because food remains in your stomach for two, three or four hours after eating, your stomach will tell you how suitable that food is. If you feel comfortable, it is likely the food you've eaten is harmonious. However, you will often feel heavy, lethargic and dull after eating, with a real sense of 'over-fullness'. Here the message is clear. Eat less. On other occasions, you might experience a queasy feeling in the stomach, a sick feeling, or the pains of indigestion. Gas or flatulence is common, too, and you need to discover what it is you are eating that creates this discomfort. Samuels and Bennett in *The Well Body Book*, suggest you mentally go down a list of the foods you have just eaten, asking yourself or your stomach whether any of them is the cause of your complaint. They claim that, with practice, you'll feel a change in the sensations in your stomach at thought of the offending food. I'd suggest the pendulum as an alternative approach to help you locate the source of your problem.

Jocelyn checks her food with the pendulum but she rarely suffers any discomfort from the food she eats. Most of her meals comprise foods in their natural states, such as raw fruit and vegetables, seeds, nuts and wholegrains. Her red meat intake is limited to three times a week, with perhaps veal on another occasion. However, she does like white meat, eating a lot of fish and poultry. No fluid accompanies her meals, though she usually drinks decaffinated coffee or fruit juice about an hour before eating. The salt shaker and the sugar bowl are conspicuous by their absence, and Jocelyn eats very sparingly of pastries, pies, packaged cereals and biscuits. Rarely does she eat fried foods, and then only using a low fat oil such as safflower oil or a non-stick pan without additional oil. More frequently, however, she grills or steams her food.

FOOD SUPPLEMENTS

Following the advice of Paavo Airola, one of the world's leading nutritionists, she uses various *food supplements* to round out her diet. *Brewer's yeast*, possibly the best source of the B complex vitamins as well as a source of protein, is usually taken as a between meals snack with fruit juice or yoghurt. Many people take a tablespoon or two a day of this food supplement but Jocelyn uses only two teaspoonsful a day, being aware of its tendency to raise the uric acid level of the blood. Because it contains no sugar and starches, Brewer's yeast is an excellent component of a reducing diet.

Cod liver oil is another of her valued supplements, taken primarily for its vitamin A, D and F content. Fresh *raw wheat germ* provides Jocelyn's main source of Vitamin E, although it also contains Vitamin B complex, protein, unsaturated fatty acid, minerals and enzymes. Obviously, wheat germ is a most valuable food.

So, too, is *kelp* which is taken regularly with her meals as a source of iodine, minerals and trace elements. Actually, Jocelyn takes most of her supplements with her meals, including *bone meal* for its mineral content, *whey powder*, which is rich in lactose, minerals, iron and the Vitamin B complex, and *rose hips* for its Vitamin C, bio-flavinoids and enzymes. Bio-flavinoids, of which family ascorbic acid is only one member, do seem to provide some immunity against allergies if taken regularly.

You will probably have noticed that Jocelyn takes her supplements in their natural form rather than as synthetically formulated vitamin and mineral pills. This is another important nutritional principle. In nature, vitamins and minerals are not isolated, being present always in the form of complexes. Thus, when vitamin and mineral supplements are taken as natural unprocessed foods, it ensures that all nutritive factors are present in their appropriate balanced combination, so the body can assimilate them effectively.

Unlike Jocelyn, most of us take our supplementary vitamins and minerals in pill or tablet form. This procedure does have the disadvantage that the chemically synthesized vitamins and minerals exist in isolation, perhaps lacking other elements not yet recognized as important to their action. Therefore, whenever possible, it does seem desirable to take our supplements in natural form. Obviously this is impossible when massive doses of vitamins are required, especially Vitamins B and C. However, even under these circumstances, it is advisable to combine the synthetic vitamin with its natural counterpart. For example, should you require large doses of synthetic Vitamin B complex, take yeast at the same time. If C is the vitamin in question, combine it with fruit juices and rose hips.

IMPORTANCE OF GOOD EATING HABITS

Not only does Jocelyn, who is now appearing somewhat as a paragon of virtue, eat nutritionally sound food, she also practices good eating habits. Firstly, she eats only when she is hungry and drinks only when she is thirsty. Sounds obvious doesn't it? Yet many of us eat because the clock tells us it is time to eat, not because our bodies need nourishment. This is a point to be elaborated in the next chapter on weight control. It is particularly important in the face of expert advice to eat a big breakfast containing a variety of foods to provide essential nutrients. This advice might be suitable for some people, but many of us simply do not feel hungry first thing in the morning. *Your* food and drink requirements are likely to be different from those of other people, so listen to your body's signals. One of the best ways of ensuring longevity and good health well into old age is to systematically undereat. This is difficult to do if you eat because the clock tells you to do so rather than because your body indicates its need for food.

Unlike the common 'food-bolter', Jocelyn eats slowly in a relaxed, unhurried atmosphere. If she is upset, angry, or disturbed, she simply does not eat at that time. Negative emotions interfere with digestion and certainly remove the pleasure from eating.

Eating slowly, too, is very important for it allows food to be broken down in the mouth. Careful chewing ensures that only pieces of manageable size, thoroughly mixed with saliva, go down to the stomach. Enzymes can then reach every fibre of the food, resulting in rapid digestion in the stomach. According to Dr Donald Norfolk in *The Habits of Health*, thorough chewing of food protects our teeth, through stimulating the flow of saliva. This helps flush away food particles adhering to the teeth. When we chew foods like carrots and apples, the small fibrous particles released act like dental floss, cleaning between teeth. Bad breath, bleeding gums and decaying teeth are all likely to improve when you chew your food thoroughly, and, by so doing, increase circulation.

Because she is not tied to the clock, and eats when she feels the need, Jocelyn tends to have several small meals during the day, perhaps as many as five or six. She feels better on this regime than on one in which she eats fewer large meals. In the past, these have left her feeling bloated, gassy and 'overfull'. Also, with these small meals, Jocelyn tries to avoid mixing too many foods. Many nutritional experts claim that each food requires a different enzyme system, and the fewer foods you mix at any one meal, the better your digestion and assimilation will be. In particular, some people experience stomach discomfort if they mix raw fruits and raw vegetables at the same meal, or take fruit and milk together. Starches such as cereals, spaghetti and potatoes frequently produce flatulence if eaten with fruit. Again, it is a matter of you finding out for yourself which foods you can safely mix.

The observant reader may have noticed that Jocelyn's habit of taking numerous small meals during the day contradicts one of the basic health rules given in Chapter Two. It was there suggested that you eat three regular meals a day without between meal snacks. However, this book espouses the philosophy that rules are made to be broken if they do not seem to suit you. Three regular meals a day did not suit Jocelyn as well as more frequent small snacks. This is true, also, for many people trying to lose weight. Rules are for guidance. They should not become straitjackets.

There are several points not stressed in the description of Jocelyn's eating habits which round out the picture of sound nutrition.

- Foods which are free of chemicals such as sprays and preservatives are probably more healthful for you than those which contain chemicals. Despite assurances to the contrary, we just do not know the effects when these substances are added to our food.
- Coffee should be taken in moderation, if at all. For many people, the caffeine in even a single cup of coffee is sufficient to bring on anxiety symptoms. The problem is compounded if cola drinks, cocoa, and chocolate-flavoured foods are also taken. These increase the caffeine intake. Caffeine would seem to have addictive properties and, in combination with nicotine, alcohol and refined sugar, puts a tremendous strain on the body's ability to control blood glucose levels. Some nutritionists would argue that many of our emotional disturbances are a result of this combination.

Cheraskin and Ringsdorf, the two doctors who wrote the book *Psychodietetics*, have claimed that emotional problems can be prevented, treated, and cured by improved nutrition. They see food nutrients as the key to emotional health, doing more to combat all known ailments than any miracle drug, and would support a diet based on meat, eggs, poultry, fish, whole grain cereals, fresh fruits, nuts, seeds, dairy products and fresh vegetables. Avoidance of refined carbohydrates, sugar, white flour foods, desserts, starchy sweets, fast foods, and sweetened drinks is the other side of the coin. So, hopefully, if you choose to change your eating pattern to that outlined in this section, your emotional health is likely to improve as markedly as your physical health. Perhaps the irritability, restlessness, depression, anxiety, and nervous breakdown which is so much a part of everyday life is a function of our diet. Change the diet and change the person.

There is no *single* food which will create this miracle of change, though, in the next section, we will be looking at some foods which do have properties of great value. Neither is there any small group of foods which contain every nutritional element which is necessary for good health. *Variety* is the key, for our bodies require many nutrients which work in combination. These your body will receive if you are guided by the principles of this section. As an old Chinese proverb has it, when you eat, the first eight parts are for you, and the last two parts for the doctor. If your last two parts are primarily composed of sugar, salt, animal fats and highly processed food, you are aggravating your health problems.

FOODS OF SPECIAL VALUE

Though there exists no single miracle food, some do figure more prominently than others in the writings of nutritional experts. Some of these, such as brewer's yeast, wheat germ, and cod liver oil have been mentioned already.

In *The Natural Health Book*, Sydney nutritionist Dorothy Hall simplifies the issue of vitamins by saying: 'If you eat wheatgerm, yeast, fresh green vegetables and fresh fruits, and vegetable oils and some oils from fish, you should be getting sufficient vitamins.'

However, Dorothy Hall, in company with other nutritionists, sees great value in foods such as honey, garlic, kelp, yoghurt, sprouts, parsley and potatoes. I would suggest you read her excellent book for its detail on individual foods and their contribution to your health.

Parsley, for example, is a most powerful and concentrated source of vitamins and minerals. One of its particularly valuable attributes is that, if eaten together with meat, it helps the system rid itself of the excess uric acid produced when the meat is digested. This is important, for arthritis, rheumatism, kidneystones, gout and gallstones can all be aggravated by such excess.

Parsley is not the only way of coping with this problem.

Reducing meat intake to no more than three or four times a week is another preventative. The protein thus lost from the diet can be replaced by beans, peas, lentils and *nuts*. Nuts such as almonds, pecans, and walnuts provide an excellent meat substitute for they do not contain uric acid, and their end products do not break down into uric acid. Grapes are another food, valuable for the elimination of uric acid from the system and for re-establishing the appropriate acid-alkaline balance of the body. Potatoes, too, achieve the same end.

Potatoes are, in fact, a much maligned food because of the unfounded fear that they are extremely fattening. Actually, potatoes are eighty per cent water and contain only one-third as many calories as an equivalent weight of bread. Especially if cooked in their skins, potatoes are an important source of vitamin C and of iron, and if grated, may be used most effectively as a poultice for infections, bites and skin irritations.

A number of foods have a natural laxative effect, providing a much safer way of combating the problem of constipation than through the use of purgatives. Some of the best known of these foods are prunes, dates, figs, citrus fruits, apples, grapes, peaches, green vegetables, olives, walnuts, berries, onions and yoghurt. From this list, it would seem clear that a fruit diet would be an excellent treatment for constipation. The added benefit would be its low calorie content, a fact of interest to those wanting to lose weight. It is the high fibre content of fruit which gives its laxative properties, another reason why it should be eaten raw. *Bran*, too, may be used to combat constipation for the same reason. Addition to the daily diet of two tablespoons of bran is a most effective way of both improving bowel function and of absorbing fewer kilojoules into the body, again of interest to weight watchers. A fruit not mentioned earlier, the *banana*, is particularly interesting in that it functions as a regulator of the large intestine. Thus it can be of value in treating both constipation and diarrhoea.

Garlic is another food which functions in this way, aiding both digestion and bowel functions. Actually garlic is much prized as a vegetable antibiotic for, when crushed, it is a powerful antiseptic. During both World Wars, military doctors, forced to improvise, used it to prevent septic poisoning and gangrene. It has also been widely employed for cystitis, sinusitis, bronchitis, gastritis and to lower blood pressure. Used in food, it has value as an illness preventative, while, in cases of infectious disease, large doses of up to twenty garlic oil capsules a day have been used. The disadvantage with garlic is the smell, offensive to many people. Chewing parsley or a few roasted coffee beans after taking may help to alleviate this problem. Age old remedies for relieving colds usually include garlic, one of the most effective being to hold a cut clove on either side of the mouth between the teeth and the cheeks. An additional benefit of this method is it is said to help teeth root more firmly. Applied to pimples, garlic will frequently help them disappear and, taken internally and applied externally, it has been found quite beneficial for rheumatic sufferers. Generally then, garlic is well worthy of inclusion in the diet on a regular basis.

So, too, is *yoghurt*. If garlic, as a natural antibiotic, does not cope with your infection and you have to turn to medically prescribed antibiotics, it is advisable to eat yoghurt at the same time. Antibiotic drugs destroy the infection producing bacteria in your system but tend to make a clean sweep in so doing, removing the friendly bacteria as well. Yoghurt will replace these and protect you against the illnesses which often strike the body left relatively unprotected after a course of antibiotics. Because it contains live bacterial culture and live enzymes, yoghurt assists proper digestion and elimination, increasing your resistance to infection as it does so. It has also been found of value in cases of stomach ulcers and, should you have wined and dined too freely, it is a good choice for breakfast the following morning.

Honey, in combination with Vitamin C, has always had its supporters as a 'hangover' remedy as well as being of undoubted value as an alleviator of cold symptoms. It is valued as a bacteria fighting agent of use in the treatment of wounds. With infected fingers, where pus has gathered, honey poultices have been used with some success. Like foods mentioned earlier, honey is a natural laxative. In addition it possesses sedative value, relieving stomach ulcers, soothing jangled nerves and assisting insomniacs to sleep. Because it can be so quickly and easily assimilated into the body, honey is an ideal source of fast energy, and it is accordingly prized by athletes. Its vitamin and mineral content is quite high, the darker it is, the more minerals it contains.

Kelp, as previously mentioned, is another food of great value as a supplement being, as it is, an extremely rich source of minerals and vitamins. Dorothy Hall often prescribes it for patients with stubborn, vague symptoms which have proven resistant to other forms of natural treatment, adding the caution that it may be some weeks before benefits become noticeable.

JUICES—VEGETABLE AND FRUIT

This may also be true of *vegetable juice treatments*. Occasionally rapid results are obtained, but it is more usual for vegetable juices to produce a slow, steady improvement in health. John Battersby is a man who has included vegetable juices as a significant element of his diet for many years. Basically he relies upon *carrot juice*, high in vitamins B, C, D, E, G and K, which he consumes at a rate of one litre a day. Experts consider that to derive any real benefit from vegetable juice therapy, a person needs to consume at least half a litre a day. Fortunately, John enjoys carrot juice, believing it to be excellent as a body cleaner. It also has undoubted benefits in eye and skin problems.

Supporters of vegetable juice therapy point to the way in which the fresh juice is converted to body energy fifteen minutes after being taken. Thus they see it as a rapid power source. Whether this is actually true or not, many people claim to feel far healthier once they add vegetable juice to their diet. John's wife, Pam, for example, adds *alfalfa* to the carrot juice, believing this combination to have been particularly beneficial in clearing up the lung problems of her youth. She has also encouraged her son to use this combination, affirming it 'cured' his sinusitis after all else failed. This seems quite likely as alfalfa is a rich source of chlorophyl and a drop of chlorophyl up each nostril night and morning is an excellent remedy for sinus headaches.

Another widely used combination is *asparagus*, *beet*, *carrot* and *cucumber*, said to aid sufferers with rheumatism, neuritis and prostate troubles. *Cabbage* juice is much prized as a nerve tonic, particularly by insomniacs. Blended with *carrot* and *celery* juice it acts as a curative agent for asthma and hay fever. When carrot and celery juice are combined with *potato* juice, benefits are derived by those suffering from gout and sciatica. The *spinach-carrot* blend is considered highly as a general health drink, *parsley* juice helps women with menstrual irregularity, and *lettuce* juice is said to act as a muscle and hair restorer. Despite doubts raised over such claims, it is incontestible that many people have benefited greatly through adding raw vegetable juices to their diet. You, too, may find the addition helpful, even if it involves only drinking the water in which your vegetables are cooked, for valuable mineral salts are contained therein.

Fruit juices, too, have their adherents, though it is generally considered better to eat the whole fruit. When suffering from a cold, for instance, it is preferable to eat lemons or oranges because it is the white pith just beneath the skin which actually contains the bioflavinoid substances. However, there is considerable evidence that *lemon juice* mixed with hot water is beneficial for sore throats, colds, influenza, dyspepsia, and stomach upset generally. *Pineapple juice*, too, is valuable, containing as it does enzymes which destroy many kinds of acute infections. Pam Battersby, referred to earlier, has used it with two of her children as an aid in healing abscesses and boils. Her mother, from whom Pam derived much of her interest in juice treatments, makes an energizer every day comprising three cups of water, one cup of honey, two cups of orange juice and two cups of grape juice blended together. Perhaps it is the secret of her vitality for at eighty-seven she is an extremely active, bright person. Another of her favourite drinks is *mineral water*, created by juicing *watermelon rind* to make an alkaline drink.

SPROUTS

Although professional nutritionists may occasionally argue over the relative merits of various vegetable and fruit juices, they are unanimous in extolling the virtues of *sprouts*. When seeds such as wheat, mustard, soy, alfalfa and mung beans are sprouted, their nutritional value is greatly increased. Vitamins, minerals, protein and enzymes exist in abundance, contributing, no doubt, to sprouts' reputation as excellent healing agents. Fortunately, for such health giving foods, sprouts are very easy to grow and they taste delightful.

Many methods, all of them simple, may be employed to sprout seeds. One of the most common is to place two tablespoons of the seeds in a litre-sized jar which is then filled with water. After soaking overnight, the seeds are well rinsed and left in the glass jar without water. The mouth of the jar is covered with cheesecloth held in place by an elastic band. Each day rinse the seeds three or four times. In several days, the actual time varying according to the seeds used, the sprouts are ready for eating. Sunflower seeds, for example, take two to three days whereas soy beans take four or five days. When the seeds are fully sprouted to a length of ½–1 centimetre they may be eaten or, with the top of the jar replacing the cheesecloth, stored in the refrigerator for later use. Although very tasty when eaten alone, sprouts may be mixed with other foods, particularly salads, to produce delicious results. If you prefer your sprouts in liquid form, they are delightful if blended with various vegetable juices.

There are so many good foods, foods which promote superior health, yet we so easily turn to the highly refined vitamin- and mineral-lacking products of our, perhaps, over-civilized society. Much of the food we eat does not provide the nutrients necessary for good health, yet we are either unaware of how much better food is available, or are unwilling to try more natural foods because of conditioned eating habits. In situations where we are trying to lose weight, the deficiency-of-nutrients problem is increased because so many diets advocate elimination of particular foods. This unbalancing effect is considered in the chapter on weight control.

10. Weight Control

THE PROBLEM OF OVERWEIGHT

Maureen Sayers is twenty kilos overweight—and has the theory to explain why. 'I can't help being fat. It's hereditary. Both my mother and father are big people, very much overweight. Their parents are too. What hope have I got. It runs in the family.' This sort of genetic theory is a popular one because it shifts the responsibility from the overweight individual to factors over which she has no control. Occasionally it might even be true—but only occasionally. Usually the reason for overweight has nothing to do with heredity. It is simply that the family as a whole eats too much. Probably the family cat and dog are overweight too. So it will help our discussion of the weight problem if we start from the realization that it stems from our eating more food than we need.

How do you know whether you are overweight? Usually this is no problem, but there are several simple tests you can perform to find out. Obviously you can weigh yourself and compare the results with a table showing the ideal weight for a person of your height and age. The pinch test is popular, too. Grasp a fold of skin from the centre of your body midway between the navel and groin. If this fold is thicker than your middle finger (for men) or thumb (for women) you have more weight on your body than desirable. Alternatively, you can find a book which is exactly 2.5 cm thick and become acquainted with its feel between the thumb and index finger. Folds of flesh at the side of the abdomen, waist, thigh, buttocks and the back of the arm are then held between the thumb and finger to test thickness. At no point should this thickness be more than 2.5 cm, according to the author of *Total Fitness*, Laurence Morehouse.

Assuming you realize you are overweight, your thoughts probably turn to dieting. You have no lack of material, for new weight-reduction proposals flood the market, each one extolling its claims to be *the* answer. Yet, there are dangers, quite serious dangers, involved in many such diets. Medical experts frequently issue warnings on the physical health hazards risked by people who diet indiscriminately. These include heart disease, arthritis, kidney failure and disorders of the gall bladder. Less often we hear about the emotional problems attendant on dieting, yet these are likely to be more common. Depression, anxiety, insomnia and irritability are all frequent 'side-effects' when one diets drastically.

This is probably due to the fact that not only does the dieter feel deprived, but he or she also is likely to be lacking some of the vitamins, minerals and essential trace elements necessary for the maintenance of physical and mental well-being. Most adult diets which drop below 8400 kilojoules are at risk in this respect. Yet the majority of diets recommend intakes well below this level. Many, too, concentrate on severely limiting the type of food eaten. These certainly work for a while, and weight is lost, but at the cost of mental tranquillity and, perhaps, physical harmony. The Grapefruit Diet, the Bananas and Milk Diet, the Pumpkin-Carrot Diet are examples of this approach to weight loss and no matter how good they are as foods, they cannot hope to supply all the nutrients required by the human body. Their action is to aggravate previously existing metabolic inbalances and perhaps cause other imbalances to appear.

Particularly vulnerable is the 'yo-yo' dieter, the person who puts on weight, crash-diets to reduce, and bounces right back again once the diet has finished. Emotional and physical health is endangered both while losing and gaining weight in such a situation, for crash dieting is quite dangerous. In *How to be Your Own Doctor (Sometimes)*, Sehnert quotes Dr Morton Glenn, a past president of the American Nutrition Association:

> A crash diet, by definition, is an overwhelmingly quick way to lose weight . . . Giving someone a crash diet is the equivalent of telling your daughter, "If you're late for an appointment, don't bother looking at the traffic lights."

A sensible diet plan, in Sehnert's view, is one which aims at losing about one kilo a week. Anything promising more than that ranks as a crash diet.

Why do we undertake crash diets? Probably because we feel uncomfortable as we are. John Baltimore did. Although he was only about fifteen per cent over his desired weight, John tended to tire easily. His breathing became laboured very quickly when he undertook any exercise such as climbing stairs. He had occasional pain and swellings in his joints, together with indigestion, headaches and constipation. These symptoms, all so common in our society, may not have been due solely to the extra weight John carried around each day. However, Professor John Yudkin of London University has claimed that the overweight person is more prone to such symptoms than his slimmer brethren.

John's problem, like that of many others, is that he eats more than he needs. His is a sedentary job, a paymaster at a large factory, and he takes little physical exercise, preferring to drive rather than walk. Possessing a 'sweet tooth', possibly a harmless sounding label for sugar addiction, John eats a lot of confectionery, cakes, biscuits and starches. Calorie-rich cola is his favourite drink. Being a polite man he finds it hard to resist second and third helpings of dessert at dinner parties, and extra rounds of drinks after work with his friends. Often, then John actually eats rich food and drinks alcohol when he doesn't really feel like it. If he is to avoid obesity, he will have to impose some self-discipline so that he eats when *he* feels the need of food and not when others think he should eat.

Actually John did realize the problem he was creating for himself, so he established a healthier pattern of eating and exercising for he was aware that crash diets, drugs, slimming garments and belt massagers are not the answers to overweight. As well as modifying his food intake, mainly through cutting down on starches and increasing his intake of relatively nonfattening foods such as vegetables and fruits, he took more exercise through walking and cycling. Still, John didn't spoil his enjoyment of life through taking his health regime too seriously. He still derived great pleasure from his after work drinks and from the desserts he ate at dinner parties. However, he now ate and drank when he felt like it, not when other people felt he should do so. A sensible man, John, he did not fall into the trap of making his life a misery through becoming *overly-conscious* of the food he ate and the relation it bore to his health.

SOME SUGGESTIONS ON WEIGHT CONTROL

John moved to a position of 'moderation in all things' in the steps he took to improve his eating habits. Thus, he did not adopt the popular 'magic foodstuffs' approach mentioned earlier when a few foods work the 'miracle' of weight loss. He was fully aware of the dangers of an unbalanced diet. However, he did change his behaviour in certain ways to make it easier for him to control his eating habits more effectively than he had done in the past.

He asked his wife, Elizabeth, to buy fewer cakes and biscuits. Those she did buy, or make herself, she kept out of sight. In other words, it required some degree of effort for John to get these starchy foods. Further, he rose from the table immediately he completed his meal and busied himself well away from the dining room and kitchen. In the past, John had tended to sit on after the meal, nibbling on potato crisps and biscuits. When he did feel like a snack, John made himself wait at least ten minutes before eating, to ensure he really was hungry rather than responding to a random thought. Then, he often deliberately ate something that was not one of his favourite foods.

A final behavioural change was, at mealtime, to concentrate exclusively upon his food instead of reading or watching television as had been his wont in his overweight days. By doing this, John made eating a 'pure' experience, unassociated with other events. He broke the connection between television and food and found, to his delight, that he no longer became hungry watching programmes. Simple changes really, but ones which made it easier for John to shed his excess kilos.

Considerable disagreement exists about the best way of scheduling meals. Traditionally, advice on losing weight is to eat three regular meals a day, each one providing approximately one third of our calorie needs, and to eliminate between meals snacks. Sometimes such a regime is effective but for many people it just does not seem to work.

Joan Ferguson found no difficulty in going light on food during the day but tended to eat a large evening meal with numerous snacks until bedtime. According to traditional theories of weight management, such a regime is all wrong. Snacks at night are supposed to put on more weight than ones taken earlier in the day, just as eating most of our food in one large meal is a more fattening pattern than dividing it equally between the three meals. However, Joan's experience is a very common one, and, when she attempted to lose weight, she simply could not adapt to the three even meals a day schedule.

It is the old story we have seen so often in this book, an attempt to force everyone into a single 'right' pattern. People are not like that, for they need to find the eating schedule that is 'right' for them in that it enables them to control their weight while remaining mentally content.

Although Joan was uncomfortable with the three regular meals schedule, she was able to adopt a 'little and often' policy, similar to Jocelyn's eating pattern, and had six meals or snacks during the day. Incidentally, it is interesting the way we label some things eaten as snacks, which are somehow rather 'sinful', and other things as meals which are 'good'. Joan used this labelling idea to help her, believing that a thing is what you call it. To her, snacks were 'light' whereas meals were 'heavy' comprising at least two courses. So by calling all her eating snacks she did not eat heavily at any time. What she was doing by her frequent snacks was to use her body's metabolic system to help her lose weight.

After you eat food, your metabolic system speeds up for about an hour to help you digest it more rapidly. Therefore, through eating on six occasions instead of three, Joan doubled the time her body was on 'faster burn-up'. She actually increased this already faster metabolic rate by exercising, whenever possible, during this after-food hour. Exercise raises our metabolic rate, not only during the period of activity, but also for some time afterwards. Joan walked, skipped, or did some energetic housework as soon as she had eaten, so she really helped her body burn off unwanted weight.

There were a number of other things Joan did, all of which contributed to a gradual weight loss. One was to drink liquids like water, lemon tea and dandelion coffee which are virtually calorie free. Another was to use smaller plates so she felt she was actually eating more than she was. Psychological needs can be very important and it is our perception of things, the way we see them, that is more important to us than the way things actually are. Occasionally, when particularly hungry, Joan turned to yeast which is an excellent appetite suppressant. Two teaspoons stirred into fruit or vegetable juice and taken fifteen minutes before a meal makes it far easier to eat sparingly.

Finally, Joan ate slowly and chewed her food thoroughly, behaviour which is very important if weight loss is the desired aim. Apparently it takes approximately twenty minutes for the stomach's messages of 'fullness' to reach the hypothalamus in the brain. If we bolt our food we are likely to continue eating after the stomach is replete. Eating more slowly allows time for the brain to realize we do not need additional food, which may then be left on the plate. Some of us, trained to clean up our plates completely, might feel guilty about this, but it is a guilt best overcome, for it will keep you eating food you do not need.

Joan's reorganization of her eating schedule achieved her goal of weight loss without damaging her physically or upsetting her emotionally. It suited her. However, her pattern did not suit her neighbour Shirley Jamieson, who found it too slow. She wanted more rapid weight loss and tried fasting.

FASTING

Fasting has been suggested as one solution to the mind-body

conflict which rages when we diet, or more precisely, when we crash diet. The difficulty with such diets is that we do not stick to them. The mind thinks it is a good idea to lose weight but the body objects to being deprived of certain foods. This struggle makes life miserable, and leads to early rejection of the diet.

When we fast, be it for one day or one week, we know we will eat nothing at all. The interesting thing is that usually after the first day or two, doing without food is no hardship. We just do not feel hungry. That is what Shirley found, much to her delight. Heeding the warnings about fasting, Shirley consulted her doctor before beginning. This is a wise procedure, particularly for fasts which are to last longer than forty-eight hours. A single day fast probably would not require such a consultation but this is a personal decision for you to make.

Should your health be poor, it is even more necessary to seek medical advice before embarking on a fast. Ill people *may* be at risk when they fast although, should the period of abstinence from food be coupled with adequate rest, they are likely to promote healing rather than impede it.

Initially, Shirley intended to fast over a weekend, believing, as a result of the material she had read, that weight loss for this period would be 4.5 kg. A single day fast would have shed about two kilos and Shirley wanted to lose more weight than this. However, after the weekend, Shirley felt no hunger and decided, as a result of further consultation with her doctor, to continue for a week. The result was nine kilos weight loss, together with a feeling of well being and increased energy.

Though I prefer a far more gradual weight loss regime myself, many people who have tried fasting are lavish in their praise. They feel the regime helps alleviate skin complaints, solves the constipation problem, cures respiratory problems such as asthma and hay fever, heals peptic ulcers, and relieves the symptoms of arthritis. Claims have also been made that periodic fasting slows down the aging process, for waste matter which has accumulated in the body is removed.

That is actually the theory upon which the procedure is based. The energy which is normally used by the body to digest food is released to clear waste matter and toxins from the body.

This material is eliminated through the skin, lungs, bowels and kidneys. Sometimes so much poisonous material is released in this way that a first-time faster can become quite ill, and have to end his fast prematurely. In such a case, several short fasts might be needed to 'purify' the body.

Shirley quite liked the idea of 'purification', and certainly enjoyed better health after her week's experience. She ended her fast correctly by maintaining a light diet for the next seven days, a time equivalent to the time spent fasting. Unlike some people, who practise juice fasting, Shirley lived on water only. When she broke her fast, she drank only fruit juice on the next day, gradually adding fruit, vegetables, nuts and grains until she returned to a more normal diet at the end of the second week. She was careful to avoid fat for several days after finishing her fast.

Though she was delighted with her weight loss, the aspect of her fast that most pleased Shirley was the unforced change that took place in her diet. Consciously, she made no real effort to adopt a healthier diet, but she found that sugars and starches no longer had the same appeal for her as they had in her pre-fast days. In fact, overall, she seemed to require less food. This is something that many fasters remark upon, that the body, once cleared of its accumulated waste material, appears to function better, being more selective about food, and needing less to achieve the same nutritional level.

Shirley was sensible in that the week she fasted was one in which she had no pressing commitments. She could take things easily, probably a wise precautuion if your fast is to be more than a few days. However, for short fasts of one or two days, life can continue as normal. Many people, in fact, do fast one day a week as a regular regime, with perhaps one longer fast over a holiday period. They believe fasting contributes to longevity because it is a way of life in which systematic undereating is practised.

A PLAN FOR GRADUAL WEIGHT LOSS

If fasting does not appeal to you as a means of losing weight and you have taken to heart the warnings on crash dieting, perhaps the plan suggested by Morehouse, Director of the Human Performance Laboratory of the University of California, in his book, *Total Fitness*, will be of interest. He suggests you set out to lose 14 700 kJ a week, which corresponds to a weekly weight loss of half a kilo. This you achieve by reducing your daily food intake by 840 kJ and expending 1260 kJ in physical exercise.

As far as the exercise is concerned, an hour's brisk walk will burn up 1260 kJ. Energetic dancing for an hour achieves almost as good a result, while tennis, bicycling, swimming or jogging should burn more than this target. The 'diet' side of your programme means that you simply eliminate that extra slice of bread or a biscuit or two during the day. Obviously you can adjust things so that on days you exercise very vigorously you may wish to have the extra slice while on days you do not exercise, you will eliminate 2100 kJ from your food intake.

This is a very gentle approach to weight loss and therein lies its chief merit. It is one which imposes no real physical or emotional pressure so you should be able to remain your normal cheerful self as the kilos gradually melt away. Morehouse suggests you keep a chart, weighing yourself each morning to check on your progress. The problem with this is that our weight tends to fluctuate from day to day due to weather changes, fluid retention and, in a woman's case, the stage of her menstrual cycle.

As an alternative to this daily weigh-in, I suggest you use your scales only once a week. Weigh nude before breakfast on the same day each week and keep a record of your weight, comparing it with your target. Assuming you began your reduction programme on a Monday, you would enter in a diary notebook:

Target Weight: 70 kg. Actual Weight: 70 kg. You would then enter your target weight for each succeeding Monday. The next one would be 69.5 kg, the one after 69 kg, and the one after that 68.5 kg. So, as each Monday comes around you would compare your actual weight with your target weight. Your weight is likely to fluctuate somewhat but the basic trend should be averaging half a kilo a week. If you are losing faster than that, ease up a little; if you are losing more slowly, cut out a little more food or increase your exercise.

Morehouse uses pounds rather than kilos and if your scales are calibrated in that measure, or you feel more comfortable with stones and pounds, by all means set your target as a one pound weight loss each week. The process continues until you reach your desired weight. This should be realistic. By that I mean, it is advisable to select a target which you were able to maintain comfortably at some not too distant time of your life, before the extra weight started to build up. Perhaps when you attain your first target you might then set up another lower one, following the same procedure of gradual reduction.

An approach to eating which is likely to help you achieve this gradual reduction is the one advocated several times earlier in this chapter. Eating three meals a day is a social habit, not a health need. Try missing meals occasionally if you are not hungry. The overweight person generally eats at the dictates of the clock and worries greatly about the terrible results if he or she should miss a meal.

Bruce Williamson was like that until, on one occasion, he was so busy closing a real estate sale that he missed his lunch. He did not realize he had done so until several hours later, and began to worry that he would feel headachy, ravenous, and tired as the afternoon wore on. Had he the time to continue fretting, no doubt he would have achieved this miserable state, but Bruce happened to be very busy that day, not arriving home for his evening meal until after seven o'clock. Much to his surprise he was no hungrier than usual, so for that day he had eaten less. He had actually missed a meal without any damaging effects.

Tentatively he tried missing more meals, particularly at breakfast time when he really never felt hungry anyway, and when he was particularly busy. That is the key of course. Keep busy at the time you would normally be eating. Quite soon Bruce adopted a rather 'so what' attitude to missing meals, and his weight started melting away. In any one week he would miss only one or two meals, but this was sufficient to achieve the half kilo weight loss which is increasingly supported as an ideal regime by many health experts.

Like Bruce you can take advantage of situations when getting food would be difficult. Maybe you are not in the business of selling real estate but there are numerous occasions when you really haven't the time to eat or when eating at a set time would be quite inconvenient. You can miss meals at such times and not even notice you have done so.

Vary your eating pattern in other ways, too, to suit your individual needs. Few meals but numerous snacks might suit you one day, while three meals might be more appropriate the next day. Some days you simply may not feel hungry. Perhaps you have a cold, or are relaxing at the beach in the sun. Make the most of such times. In short, eat when you feel hungry, and do not worry about the supposed health hazards of such behaviour. These are quite illusory, being based mainly on theories of dubious value. In Eastern Europe, for example, many peasant peoples still have a single meal each day when they finish their work in the fields. Others seem to get by very well on two meals, often living to a healthy old age which is the envy of Western tourists. So be your own expert, establish your own comfortable eating pattern, and lose weight doing so if this is what you desire.

11. Exercising to Improve Your Health

BEING SENSIBLE ABOUT EXERCISE

Exercise is good for us. Experts are virtually unanimous in extolling the merits of exercise as a means of improving our health. Physical conditioning schemes, ranging from simple injunctions to 'do more walking' to elaborate edifices involving calisthenics, muscle building exercise and strenuous aerobic type activities abound. Probably they are right. There does seem to be a definite link between taking reasonable amounts of exercise and good health. But how much is reasonable? Some of the experts would have us spending so much time exercising our bodies that we would have little opportunity to do anything else. Others are more moderate, attempting to blend exercise into people's lives without too much disruption.

Professor of exercise physiology, Laurence Morehouse, referred to in the previous chapter for his ideas on weight loss, is one such 'moderate'. He advocates an eminently sensible, gentle approach which seems well within the capabilities of those of us who wish to achieve an improved level of physical fitness. Morehouse, in his book *Total Fitness*, is adamant that we should not force ourselves into a lifestyle which creates strain. We have enough strain in our lives already without deliberately creating more through the adoption of an overly demanding exercise regime. The requirements of our job, the time schedules we have to meet, and the responsibilities of our family commitments prove a sufficient burden. Exercise, if it is to benefit our health, should equip us to cope better with everyday life, not make life more of a struggle than ever.

Bob Chancellor doubted that he could become fit again. A keen athlete at university, Bob had virtually forsaken exercise once he entered full-time practice as an accountant. That was over thirty years ago. Like so many of us, once he finished his day's work, he sat watching television, nibbling snacks. On weekends, he sometimes went out with the family, usually by car, or loafed about at home. Occasionally he did some gardening, but, more frequently, he really did little more than sit around, eat and read. In itself, there seems nothing particularly wrong with such a lifestyle if that is the way a person wants to spend his life. Though frequent pronouncements about the 'badness' of such lack of activity are designed to make us feel guilty, it seems to me that each person has the right to spend his time as he sees fit. If this choice is for doing virtually nothing as a relaxation from work problems, so be it.

Bob, however, had a problem. He was finding it difficult to work efficiently because he felt so sluggish and lethargic. Climbing stairs made his breathing uncomfortably heavy and he generally lacked zest. Bob thought that increased physical fitness might help him become more vital and alive, yet he doubted that thirty years of relative inactivity could be overcome. He was fifty-two years old, overweight, and tired. Obviously, a tremendous effort would be needed if he was to achieve anything worthwhile, and he just was not prepared to make such an effort.

Fortunately, he does not have to. Morehouse points out that a person's physical condition at any particular moment is primarily a function of what that person has done over the previous four weeks of his life. True, heredity, medical condition, and long-standing exercise habits play some part in present condition, but they are not nearly as important as the four week period. Bob, who has avoided exercise for most of his life, and who now wants to change this pattern, can virtually remake himself in the space of four weeks. Should he achieve this transformation he can, if he returns to his former pattern of inactivity, lose all his new found fitness in the next four weeks. Obviously, this one month period is crucial.

So Bob, if he wants to, can become a reasonably fit person in four weeks. How? Jogging is the 'in' exercise at the moment and people in their thousands, all over the world, are bobbing around on footpaths, roads, playing fields, and beaches. Great. But jogging is not for everyone, though you could be excused for thinking so in the face of the massive publicity it receives.

Val Donaldson believed it to be so. She took her jogging sensibly, started gently over short distances and built up gradually. The problem was, she always developed a crashing headache whenever she jogged. Val's body was telling her something, and eventually she listened. Swimming is now her exercise, and there are no headaches. Other people, when they jog, particularly on hard pavements, develop painful hips, knees, shins or ankles. Jogging is not for them.

I am not trying to criticize jogging as an exercise. It is a very good way of achieving an improved level of physical fitness—*for some people*. The important thing is for you as an individual to find an exercise you enjoy doing and one which helps you to feel better physically. Don't place too much store on the so-called 'best' conditioners. What is essential is for you to exercise your heart and lungs in a way which brings you pleasure. If you do so, you are likely to make of it a lifetime activity, whereas if you undertake a particular exercise because you are told how good it is for you, you will probably drop your 'get-fit' programme very quickly.

THE SAFEST FORMS OF EXERCISE

Possibly the safest activities for an unfit person to use in a reconditioning programme are those of a rhythmical nature. Jogging is one of these, together with walking, cycling, swimming, dancing, climbing, skipping and skiing. These are 'aerobic' activities, ones which involve the large muscles of the body, primarily the thighs, over an extended period of time. Pursuance of one or more of these means of exercise benefits the heart and lungs, increasing their capacity to process more oxygen in a given period of time. Aerobic exercises make you breathe deeply, you tend to huff and puff more than you would in a resting state, and, by so doing, take in increased amounts of air. The more you regularly exercise in this way the more your heart and lungs become capable of doing additional work, and of producing additional energy. Any activity, therefore, that causes you to breathe hard for a reasonable time is very valuable to your health.

The term 'reasonable' time is interpreted differently by different experts. Morehouse feels you need only thirty minutes a week spread over three ten-minute sessions to achieve fitness. However, he does stress that you should increase the vigour with which you perform your daily tasks and thus get more exercise this way. Others assert that fifteen minutes an exercise session five days a week is the absolute minimum with thirty minutes a session being even better. However, once you feel pressured by having to devote excessive amounts of time to your programme, you will lose the benefits. Find, through experimentation, what suits you. Personally, I lose interest if I follow an every second day exercise schedule as recommended by Morehouse. By adopting a regular routine, I do my activities as a matter-of-course, not having to think about when I am to do them. I know that every morning before breakfast I either jog, cycle, swim or skip, depending on which activity I feel like on that particular day. In fact, once you do adopt such a routine as your normal life style, you miss it should you be unable to exercise for any reason.

Though all the aerobic exercises, if engaged in on a continuous basis, will help you improve your health, perhaps walking and swimming are considered most highly as all-round conditioners for the unfit person.

Walking, with its easy flowing rhythm, has a soothing effect, easing away the worries of the day. Many married couples have found an evening walk to be an ideal way, not only of exercising, but also of improving communication between them. Problems discussed while walking have a habit of being solved rather quickly. The philosopher, Bertrand Russell, often extolled the psychological benefits of the long distance walk, believing that it was one of the best means of increasing our happiness. Deep changes in personal philosophy, he believed would be far less beneficial to unhappy businessmen than a daily ten-kilometre walk.

It is an activity that burns up the kilojoules too. Estimates vary somewhat, but it would appear that a brisk half-hour walk could remove up to 1000 kJ. Jogging or running this distance achieves the same result, for the speed at which the ground is covered is apparently irrelevant. Obviously, though, a runner who exercises for half an hour will achieve more than a walker, because he will cover a greater distance.

Walking, then, can assist you to lose weight and improve your psychological health. It can also improve the circulation of your blood, being of considerable benefit if you suffer from varicose veins and chilblains. Deteriorating circulation is often seen as a sign of aging. So, also, are stiff joints, flabby muscles and breathlessness during and after exertion. Yet these symptoms are more a function of lack of exercise than of aging, and walking will help you realize that this is so. You are likely to find you are actually younger than you previously felt you were.

Swimmers reap this benefit too. Like walking, it is an all-round exercise which conditions most muscles of the body. Unlike many other aerobic activities, swimming is easy on the legs and spine in that no jarring is involved. With the body supported by the water, the swimmer can exercise without worrying about the possible ill-effects of pounding his feet onto a hard, unyielding surface. That is, perhaps, one of the reasons why swimming, or more precisely backstroke, is such an excellent treatment for back troubles. With no jarring of his spine taking place, the swimmer literally 'massages' the damaged back area as he strokes through the water.

It is important, then, to select your own means of exercise, that which will bring you both enjoyment and fitness. It is also important to go about it in a sensible way. Murray Thomas did not. He played squash once a week 'to keep fit' but led an otherwise sedentary life. The once weekly game did little towards conditioning Murray's body, but the short bursts of intense effort imposed a tremendous strain on his heart. His pulse rate shot up alarmingly, he gasped for breath, often turning purple in the face, and he felt distressed for some time after he stopped playing. Being highly competitive, Murray played hard. He continued to do so until he dropped dead of a heart attack at forty-three. This happened in the dressing room just after he came off the court.

Murray was unwise to play so hard once a week and take virtually no exercise for the rest of the time. Yet he is certainly not alone in his folly. The weekend golfer is a perfect example. Perhaps you feel golf is too gentle a game, compared to squash, to create the same problem. It is less likely to do so, certainly, but there are numerous cases of unfit golfers being adversely affected by a hard game. Any pattern of vigorous exercise on a once-a-week basis is asking for trouble, so it would seem advisable to adopt the virtually unanimous advice of the experts on this point and to exercise on a steady, regular basis. If you do so, it becomes part of your life, conditioning you to cope with periods of more intense effort without putting dangerous pressure on yourself.

EXERCISE AND ITS BENEFITS

Sarah Hoddle is very hard headed about everything she does. That is why she runs both her home and her career as a fashion designer so successfully. Sarah always weighs advantages against disadvantages before committing herself to any line of action. As she approaches her mid-thirties, Sarah is becoming more aware of the need to improve her health. A succession of minor health problems are plaguing her. A feeling of 'never being quite well' has become her normal state. Despite taking increasing care over her diet and trying various vitamin-mineral supplements, Sarah feels something is lacking. Medical advice has not been beneficial, naturally enough, for her symptoms are rather vague. Various medications may have contributed to the healing of specific skin complaints, a sinus condition and swollen glands, but Sarah realized her problem was more general than this. As fast as one symptom improved another took its place.

Exercise and Sarah, though not enemies, could hardly be said to be friends. Sarah was always too busy to 'waste time' in this way though she did keep active around the house, and, to some extent, at work. However, her friend Evelyn, seemed to have benefited so much from her newly adopted activities of skipping and jogging, that Sarah decided to follow suit. She decided the possible advantage of improved health far outweighed the relatively slight time commitment and justified a change in her lifestyle.

Sarah started her day with a few exercises designed to increase body flexibility. She continued with five minutes skipping, a time which she increased to a maximum of ten minutes over a period of two weeks. Both these activities took place before breakfast. After her evening meal, Sarah and her husband, Don, began taking a walk of approximately 3 kilometres. This was her exercise programme, one which she has now maintained for the past two years because she found it made a positive contribution to her health. Although she still experiences the occasional ailment, no longer is she plagued by a succession of such problems. In addition, she feels better, more energetic and lively, better able to handle emergencies, less fatigued at the end of the day.

The beneficial effects Sarah derived from her exercise are rather typical. Most people delight in a new found sense of muscle awareness, of increased physical competency. This is a very enhancing feeling and does wonders for the self-concept, for the fit person believes he is more effective in handling the challenges of everyday life. When other people comment on this, too, the self-concept is further enhanced and this is what happened with Sarah. Don commented on her increased vitality and improved health, on her younger appearance. This praise provided a very positive reinforcement for Sarah to maintain her programme.

It has been theorized that continued physical activity improves body tissues and body functions, thus slowing down the aging process. There does appear to be some support for this view in studies of mortality rates. A survey of over one million men and women aged from forty-five to eighty-four indicated that, as the amount of exercise increased, so the death rate declined. In the fifty to fifty-four male age group level, for example, there were 2.08 deaths per hundred for the non-exercisers, 0.80 deaths per hundred for the slight exercisers, 0.55 deaths per hundred for the moderate exercisers, and 0.33 deaths per hundred for the strenuous exercisers.

These results were used by Cheraskin and Ringsdorf in *Psychodietics* to illustrate that the benefits of exercise and nutrition go hand in hand. Though the exercisers in the study consumed approximately the same total number of calories as did the non-exercisers, they had a higher intake of vitamins, minerals and amino acids. They also consumed far less coffee, tea, alcohol, tobacco, sugar and refined carbohydrates. Why should this be so? Cheraskin and Ringsdorf argue that exercising helps control blood-glucose levels and by doing so, helps prevent the hypoglyoaemic cycle with its craving for sweets and sugar.

Whether this theory is true or not, it does seem reasonable to accept that non-exercisers tend to overload the heart. Morehouse points out that the heart muscle and the muscles of the body are meant to work together as a mutual support system. Physical activity ensures that this occurs with the skeletal muscles becoming what they were intended to be — auxiliary hearts. When the body is relatively motionless, the heart gets no such assistance and is called upon to do extra work for which it was not designed. This view makes highly suspect, on health grounds, the constant 'keep still' injunctions of school teachers to their students. It would seem preferable for people to move around occasionally, to fidget. This ensures a more adequate blood supply to the brain, particularly when a person is in a sedentary situation for much of the day.

Exercise, then, in general terms is likely to be beneficial in prolonging life. Hopefully, it will also enable you to enjoy in better health the years you have gained. The person who is physically fit at the onset of an illness is more likely initially to offer strong resistance than one who is not. Even should he be unable to completely check this illness, he will be able to maintain his normal lifestyle for a longer period of time before succumbing. Should surgery be necessary, the exerciser is more likely to survive and recover rapidly than the non-exerciser.

Even in the sexual sphere, the regular exerciser would seem to have an advantage. There is evidence to suggest he or she is likely to maintain an active sex life for longer than his or her more sedentary peers, possibly due to the self-enhancing effect of exercise referred to earlier. It seems to be the case that a person who does not feel good about himself or herself is unlikely to send very positive sexual signals to others.

Earlier it was suggested that walking is a soothing activity. Dr Herbert de Vries of the University of Southern California has extended this view, claiming that exercise generally has a tranquilizing effect. Fifteen minutes of exercise, he believes, can alleviate short-term stress and reduce long standing nervous tension. Free of the side effects of chemical tranquilizers, exercise would seem a more desirable first step treatment of stress, calming the mind and body in a very natural way.

SETTING YOUR EXERCISE GOALS

If, like Sarah of our previous example, you are willing to try building more exercise into your lifestyle, it is worthwhile considering why you want to take such action.

Perhaps reducing tension is your goal in undertaking an exercise programme. Maybe your ill health is providing the motivation. Whatever reason or reasons you have for becoming an exerciser rather than a non-exerciser, it is important to be clear about what you are trying to do before you actually start. These goals or objectives should embrace things you enjoy doing. As stressed earlier, it is counter-productive to compel yourself to exercise more.

If you feel you are forcing yourself to exercise, I would suggest you are likely to do more harm than good because you are summoning up negative emotions. Exercise becomes equated in your mind with unpleasantness, creating a self-imposed session of misery for you each time you force yourself into action. You are depressed, irritated and angry because you are trying to make yourself keep a commitment which, in your heart, you know you are not going to honour. When, as is inevitable, you stop your exercising, you feel guilty and inadequate with a sense of having let yourself down. Who needs such a collection of negative emotions, particularly when you are generating them for yourself.

Rather, link your exercise with positive emotions, feelings of enjoyment, by setting your goal sufficiently low that you can live with it comfortably. In this way you experience success, and this encourages you, rewards you for your efforts, and maintains your exercise behaviour. The moral of the story, then, is to be content with taking a walk each day, if this is what gives you pleasure, rather than force yourself, with gritted teeth, into jogging along with a group of your neighbours.

You are the person to set your exercise goal, not someone else who purports to know what is best for you. Maybe he does, but the theme of this book is that you are likely to be the best expert on your own body and what is good for it. I say this knowing full well we insist on poisoning our bodies with nicotine, alcohol, and other drugs. Yet, most of us do this knowing we are damaging ourselves. Whether we want to accept it or not, we are making a choice. We are choosing to inflict damage on our bodies and choosing not to adopt a healthier lifestyle. No matter how many people tell you the way to best live your life, you will not follow such advice until you are ready to do so. When you are ready to take more exercise, do it in a way which makes you feel good, even if it is not the way the experts recommend.

Begin by accepting the importance, to you, of physical activity. Once you do so, you will be able to find time for it in your life. Judy Tremaine, who is a friend of my wife, is constantly saying how much she would like to do more exercise but she just does not have the time for it. What Judy is really saying is that exercise is not sufficiently important for her to make time to do it. We *always* have time for something that we see as really valuable.

Having accepted the importance of increased physical activity, make sure that you actually do create time for it. Plan for a particular time each day, or each second day, to be set aside for exercising, a time which is not to be encroached upon by any other activity. As a high priority item in your life, physical activity merits its own block of 'space'.

Finally, realize the importance of the attitude you adopt. A physical activity, skipping for example, is an event, something that happens. You can adopt a positive attitude towards this event 'I like skipping', or you can adopt a negative attitude, 'I don't like skipping'. The event itself is neutral. It does not change. Your attitude to events can and does change, and you can choose the attitude you want to adopt. The way you think about events determines whether you will enjoy them or not.

This is true for your life as a whole, a point stressed in my earlier book, *The Plus Factor*. As we grow older, we lose, to some extent, our capacity to perform, but many of us deteriorate far more rapidly than is really justified. Is our decline an inevitable result of advancing years, or is it more a function of our changed activity pattern? Because we adopt an attitude that older people engage in less physical activity, we tend to do less, thus encouraging deterioration in our capacity to perform. Through holding such an attitude, we condemn ourselves to spiral downward because, as we do less, our ability to exert ourselves decreases. Because our ability has become less, our desire for physical activity diminishes and we slide quickly into 'old age'. There is an old saying that 'if you don't use it you lose it.' Therefore, use your body, enjoy physical activity and you have an excellent chance of defying the decline attributed to aging for quite some time. It is, so much, a matter of the attitude you choose to adopt.

PULSE RATE THEORY

Often it is difficult to know whether the exercise you do is really assisting you to achieve greater fitness. The traditional measures, such as performing for a certain length of time, or over a certain distance, or under a certain physical load, are helpful but rather imprecise. For the person who wants to find out how best he can use exercise to improve his physical condition, pulse rate theory would seem to provide a reasonably convenient and accurate indicator.

My introduction to this concept took place more than ten years ago. Bob Roberts, my regular squash opponent, came out to play on one occasion and kept stopping after every long rally in order to check his pulse rate. I found this disconcerting, to say the least, as I based my game on running my opponent around the court until he tired. Obviously, I could not do this while Bob insisted on this continual monitoring of his pulse rate. He explained that his rate should not go over 180 beats a minute or else the consequences would be terrible to behold. Accordingly, when I had him nicely puffed, he would wait until his pulse rate dropped back below the danger level. Very sensible, but frustrating to me.

Since that time I have come to realize just how valuable an indicator of physiological functioning this measure is. The heart is immediately available to tell you, at any given moment, at what level your body is working. Your pulse rate indicates the speed at which your heart is beating and makes it possible for you to design an exercise programme which meets your individual needs. That is, you can decide on the distance you should cover and the speed at which you cover that distance by the effect your activity has upon your pulse rate.

As Morehouse points out, the advantage of the pulse rate as a measure of physiological response is that it is so easy to measure, summing up in a single score the relative effort expended by the various systems of the body. When Bob ran hard during long rallies, the physical effort he exerted was great, a fact reflected by his raised heart rate. When he was more in control of the rally, he needed to move but little and his pulse rate was much lower.

Generalizing this concept, it means that if, during your walk or your swim, your heart rate remains low, you are not really conditioning your body to any marked extent. To make a more positive contribution to improving your fitness, you need to increase your level of activity to a point where your pulse rate is around 120 beats a minute. On some days, when you are feeling below par, it will require relatively little effort for you to reach this level. When you are feeling fitter, more effort is needed to attain the appropriate level of activity. So it is not really the actual physical performance which is important. Rather it is the amount of effort involved, and this is what your pulse measures. Emphasis, then, shifts from the external factors of distance covered, time taken, and weight lifted to the internal factor of heartbeat.

You carry within you your own measuring device and this enables you to adjust your physical activity accordingly. Initially, you record your resting pulse rate. This you do when you are inactive, a few hours after eating, smoking or drinking. Obviously, too, you wait until you have fully recovered from any physical exertion. Should your resting pulse rate be higher than 80 beats a minute, you are likely to be both unhealthy and unfit. However, as you make your heart beat faster during short periods of exercise, your resting heart rate becomes lower. Your fitness increases and your heart performs more efficiently. The faster beat you aim for is around 120, and it is desirable to maintain that pulse rate for several minutes at a time each day. Once you attain a reasonable level of fitness you gain virtually nothing by exercising below this rate. Incidentally, when checking your pulse during physical activity to see whether you have attained the 120 beat level, keep moving around. Do not attempt to take your pulse while standing still.

This, then, could be your goal, to exercise for several minutes each day with a pulse beat of 120. By doing so, you will maintain a high level of fitness. However, should you so desire, you can go further. Your maximum heart rate is about 220 beats a minute minus your age, and you can use this figure to plan an effective conditioning programme.

Vic Houseman can serve as an example. Aged forty, Vic lived a very sedentary life, both at home and in his job as a dental mechanic. For a variety of reasons Vic decided to do something about his lack of fitness and he used pulse rate as his measuring instrument. His maximum heart rate was 180, and he began his exercising at the level of 60% of this rate, namely 108. That is, each day he jogged at such a speed that he held his pulse rate at

108 beats for seven or eight minutes. This level he maintained for two weeks, by which time he was not really extending himself at all.

Vic then moved to his next level, 70% of his maximum heart rate or 126 pulse beats a minute. Another two weeks of jogging saw him achieving this quite easily. After four weeks he had achieved quite a high level of fitness, but he wanted to go further, moving onto a pulse beat level of 144, 80% of his maximum, which he maintained for the seven or eight minute period. This was the level Vic remained at in his fitness programme, for he knew that exercising at more than 80% of his maximum heart rate would confer no additional benefit and attempting to sustain a level of 100% could be detrimental to his health. Of course, not all of us would choose to exercise at such a high level. It would depend on our goals.

STRETCHING THE BODY

To this point I have been talking about aerobic exercises, for it is those which increase the capacity of heart and lungs and produce the most obvious improvement in health. However, calisthenics have been popular for many years, mainly for their 'limbering-up' effect. Many people like to start the day flexing their muscles, loosening them after hours in bed. Others prefer to stretch their muscles in the evening. Should you wish to increase your flexibility in this way there are a number of exercise combinations which have stood the test of time.

To develop and maintain a full range of movement in all your joints, try the following exercises. Breathe easily and freely as you do them.

- With your feet wide astride, circle your arms forwards, upwards and backwards.
- Keeping your feet wide astride, and with your hands on your hips, bend your upper body from side to side.
- Bring your feet together, and alternately raise your thighs to your chest.
- Feet wide astride again, stretch your arms sideways and rotate your upper body.

- With feet remaining wide astride, reach each hand alternatively towards the opposite ankle.
- Run lightly on the spot.
- Rise on your toes and perform a full knee bend.

YOGA

Yoga asanas or body postures stress relaxation and gentleness. Straining and forcing play no part in this system which has been of benefit to mankind for over 3000 years. Hatha Yoga, the 'yoga of health' is the form of yoga most popular in the Western world and many people derive great benefit from its practice without necessarily embracing its spiritual and philosophical aspects. Yoga teachers would not approve of such a separation but again the choice is yours. Practice of the body postures alone will increase your joint flexibility, but, perhaps if you accept the more spiritual aspects too, you may also develop your mental suppleness. Yoga facilitates spinal mobility, loosening ligaments and muscles in the back. It helps combat the stiffness which is, perhaps, a function of old age but is more likely to be due to an absence of stretching exercise.

Yoga practitioners believe the asanas relax mind and body, strengthen muscles and relieve tension, thus preventing illness and creating the conditions under which your body can heal itself. To some extent this is due to the augmented flow of oxygen into the system and the elimination of carbon dioxide gas. Yoga exercises are cleansing in nature, helping promote effective digestion, improved blood circulation, and efficient removal of waste products from the body.

Should you be interested in learning this system of health improving exercise, I would suggest you do so from a qualified yoga teacher. Attempting to learn yoga from a book, while possible, is likely to produce inferior results from those gained under the guidance of an experienced tutor.

ISOMETRICS ARE USEFUL TOO

Isometrics, a form of exercise which involves tensing muscles without actual movement, is particularly valuable in situations where you are waiting with nothing to do. The exercises are easy to perform and, working as they do on the principle of overload, enlarge and strengthen muscles very quickly. Unlike the flexibility type exercises described in previous sections, isometrics are concerned primarily with strengthening muscles and improving their tone and health. Perhaps their greatest value lies in the prevention of fatigue, for they appear to restore alertness at times when, through boredom or inactivity, you feel lethargic and sluggish. The improved muscle tone they create also contributes towards improved posture, reduced flabbiness, and a more zestful approach to life. Details of specific exercises are available in books such as *The Complete Book of Isometrics* written by Vic Obeck and Ridwan Aitken.

These exercises can be performed while sitting on a chair in a waiting room, enabling you to use this time more productively; while sitting in a car at traffic lights, permitting you to get the kinks out of your muscles if you have been driving for some time; or while sitting at a desk studying. The possible situations in which they might be used are many and the benefits derived are out of all proportion to the little time actually required.

EXERCISE AS A WAY OF LIFE

The real benefits of physical activity come from making it a regular part of your life rather than as something extra added on as an afterthought. Though it is very valuable to perform certain exercises which turn, twist and stretch your body to its full range of motion, and to engage in aerobic activities which raise your heart rate to 120 beats a minute for at least three minutes every day, it is even more important to take every opportunity to build physical activity into your everyday life.

Begin your day with some deep yawning and stretching while still in bed. Really extend your muscles. In your morning shower, be vigorous in the way you soap and towel yourself. Actually, hard towelling can lift your pulse rate over 100. As you dress, deliberately balance on one leg while you put on your socks and shoes. Bend to tie shoelaces, stretch to pick up clothes you may have dropped. Do a deep knee bend or two when opportunity presents itself. At work, shun the lift or escalator and walk.

Whether at work or home, don't lie when you can sit, or sit when you can stand. Look for opportunities to exercise—a bag of groceries to lift and carry, a table to shift. When you travel by bus, get off a stop early and walk the rest of the way. Take a car only when essential, using your feet instead. Reduce television viewing and do more gardening.

Life abounds with opportunities to use our bodies more. All we need to do is take advantage of these and by so doing develop increased fitness and improved health. Exercise is preventive medicine at its best, and the brief bursts of effort you put into everyday tasks are, to some extent, more beneficial than more deliberate aerobic activity. It appears that a law of diminishing returns prevails. When exercising for several minutes you get much more out of the first minute than you do out of the last. So, many short bursts of activity are likely to produce greater benefit than a few long exercise sessions.

SOME PRECAUTIONS

When you exercise, never hold your breath and strain. To gain and maintain fitness you do not have to endure pain and exhaustion. Competition athletes might, but not you, so there is no need to strain. Warm up gradually, raising your pulse rate to 120 over a period of a minute or two. Moderation in all things applies very much to exercise, for violent, forceful stretching simply invites injury.

After exercise, cool off gradually. It is preferable to either walk around or sit quietly. Do not simply stand still as blood tends to drain from the brain, producing dizziness and light headedness. There is no need to put additional clothing on until you have cooled down. When you no longer feel hot, that is the time to put on the jacket or sweater, for keeping yourself sweaty is of no value.

Of course, many people still think it is, believing that it is very beneficial to work up a 'healthy sweat'. To this end they exercise in track suits or heavy sweaters, or sit in Turkish baths, sweating profusely. At one time it was considered a sound practice, the theory being that it was an effective way of ridding the body of its accumulated waste produces and toxins. However, it is now believed that the value of exercise is quite unrelated to the sweating which may accompany it. In fact, it is potentially harmful, for an overheated body places an overload on the heart. Further, as your body has only a certain amount of energy, it seems pointless to use a lot of this supply to rid the body of excessive heat. Stay as cool as possible as you exercise and you will derive more benefit from it.

Be sensible about your exercise. If you feel unwell, don't drive yourself into action. Some people feel so guilty about missing their jog, they stagger out and go through the motions no matter how bad they feel. Behaving like this is allowing your exercise to dominate you instead of the other way around. Use exercise as you would use homoeopathic medicines or food, as a means of preventing ill health. It is essential that you stay in control, creating a lifestyle which suits you, which brings you enjoyment, and which aids you in the enhancement of your health.

12. The Breath of Life

HEALTHY BREATHING

Yoga exercises, as stated in the last chapter, place great stress on suppleness, on loosening the muscles and ligaments of the back to combat the stiffness and immobility which results from our lack of stretching and exercise. The postures involve particular methods of breathing as well as the actual physical movements. Yoga emphasizes 'correct' breathing, seeing tremendous value in this aspect of our functioning.

A basic breathing exercise designed to move the diaphragm through its complete range, blowing out old air and drawing in new, is often used as an adjunct to the yoga corpse posture in which you lie flat on your back on the floor, arms at side with palms uppermost. Gradually raise your arms until your hands are above your head. Inhale slowly until your abdomen pushes out. Exhale slowly, lowering your arms as you do so and sucking in your abdomen until it almost touches your spine.

Simplicity itself, this exercise, and it is only one of many which are based on the assumption that it is possible to improve our health by becoming more aware of the way we breathe. Breathing exercises, whether they are yogic or derived from other sources, help to relieve muscular and mental tensions, improve posture, reduce anxiety, sharpen the sensitivity of our senses, bring additional energy into the body and increases our ability to cope with stress. In particular, there would appear to be a definite relationship between a relaxed breathing rhythm and calmness. Long, deep, slow exhalations promote a feeling of 'letting go' tensions and anxieties. So to relax, be aware of your breath as you let it go. Conversely, to draw in energy and create an invigorated feeling, focus on your inhalation which may be slow or fast, and deep. Inhalation can promote anxiety, as can holding the breath, particularly when we are thinking hard or faced with stress. By letting our breath go slowly and deeply under such circumstances, we can often relieve this anxiety. Yawning, for example, is nature's way of achieving this, producing as it does a wide swing of the diaphragm, increased oxygenation of the blood, and improved blood circulation.

Breathing is, of course, quite automatic. It is a self-regulatory process which normally works in such a way as to promote our health. Unfortunately, tension and anxiety interfere with our breathing rhythm, often creating not only physical difficulties but also mental sluggishness. Lack of oxygen, a result of bad breathing, reduces mental alertness, and produces a feeling of tiredness. This fatigue, sometimes bordering on exhaustion, is accompanied, on occasion, by depression. Obviously, then, good breathing is another important factor we must consider in our desire to prevent illness and improve our health generally.

Many of us breathe poorly. Paul Evans is not atypical in this respect. His breathing is very shallow, involving his chest and not his abdomen. Under stress, Paul tends to hold his breath. This is obvious when he drives a car. The slightest increase of tension and Paul holds his breath. Even when concentrating on a task like writing a letter, he inhibits his breathing and, in more strained circumstances such as meeting strangers at a party, Paul creates tremendous tension within himself by his shallow respiration. No wonder he is so restless and finds concentration difficult.

Paul is not really conscious of the way he is breathing and of the problems he is creating for himself. Breathing can be conscious or unconscious, of course, and if Paul chooses to take more control he can solve many of his difficulties. Deep breathing is literally a regeneration process, helping you look and feel more alive. Muscle tone improves, skin looks better, you feel more relaxed, and your body becomes warmer.

Should Paul wish to concentrate on how air comes in and

goes out of his system, not only will he help himself in these ways, he will also alleviate his greatest problem, his constant worrying over trifles. As will be explained more fully later, if you focus upon your breathing your attention is diverted from other thoughts and feelings. In this way you put a temporary stop to the nagging, irritating, mental activity which upsets you and adds to your tension.

To check on his breathing, Paul undressed and stood before a full length mirror. Standing sideways so he could see his profile, Paul observed himself breathing in his normal way. His abdomen or belly remained almost motionless, though his chest rose and fell as he filled and emptied his lungs. Yet it is important that we breathe with our abdomens if we are to feel more relaxed. Not all the time, of course. During the day, at work, chest breathing may be more appropriate, for we want to feel energetic and vigorous. However, it is valuable to practise abdominal breathing so that, for at least part of the day we can more fully oxygenate our body. Deep breathing fills both abdomen and chest. You see first the abdomen pushing out as you inhale, then the chest. As you exhale, both sink in. Paul's mirror test will give you the information on your own breathing pattern.

An alternative way to practise effective breathing begins with a full exhalation to empty lungs completely. Sounding the letter 's' after you think you have emptied them ensures you get rid of the last vestige of air. Remain empty for a moment and then, very, very slowly, allow air to flow into you. Use your imagination so that you 'see' it coming in through the soles of your feet, being drawn up through your legs, spine, neck to the top of your head. Think of the air as energy filling your entire body. Perhaps you can think of it in terms of white light, or golden, or pink. Any colour you like, really, as long as your associate it with energy filling you. Keep this luminous air within you for a comfortable period.

Pauses at the end of both inhalation and exhalation are very important, contributing to a relaxed, unforced feeling. After you pause, exhale very slowly, letting the air flow from you without strain, imagining that as it goes, it carries with it any impurity of mind and body. If you can remember to breathe in this way occasionally during the day, you will refresh and relax yourself greatly. It is also useful just before going to sleep.

BREATHING FOR ENERGY

As mentioned earlier, the emphasis falls upon drawing in breath when you want to energize your body. Though the actual breathing process itself is the basic element in achieving this, its effect is increased greatly if you use your imagination too. One of the simplest, yet most effective, ways of doing so is to imagine that, as you breathe in, you are raising a column of light up from the small of your back, bringing it gently up your spine to your head, and breathing it out through your forehead.

Another imaginative exercise involving visualization of your breath as light is to see a light source directly above and in front of you. As you breathe in, you feel energy flowing into you from this source which is shining on your forehead. Your whole body is filled with this invigorating light, you glow with it. Then, as you exhale, you 'see' it flowing out through your finger tips, taking with it all tension.

The storage battery concept can be helpful, too. As you inhale, you imagine you are plugged into a battery which is charging your whole body with energy. This is a useful technique to use when you wake in the morning. Extending this imaginative idea a little, you can actually locate the battery in your solar plexus area. Its position is illustrated on page 192.

Because of the network of nerve fibres which exist at this point, it is an excellent location to imagine for the storage and conservation of energy. As you inhale, imagine charging the battery, seeing it glow with power. While exhaling, you can either leave the battery fully charged or 'see' the energy being sent to particular areas of the body which require invigorating.

Alternatively, the idea of building a reservoir of energy might appeal to you more. A popular location is in the region of the navel. Another is in the chest area. Energy is drawn in during inhalation and stored in the reservoir, where it glows within you, ready to be used for emergencies. A useful device which can be used at such times is to use a pump image. To draw energy from the reservoir imagine, as you inhale, that you are lifting the handle of a pump. As you exhale, imagine pumping the energy to the part of the body which requires it.

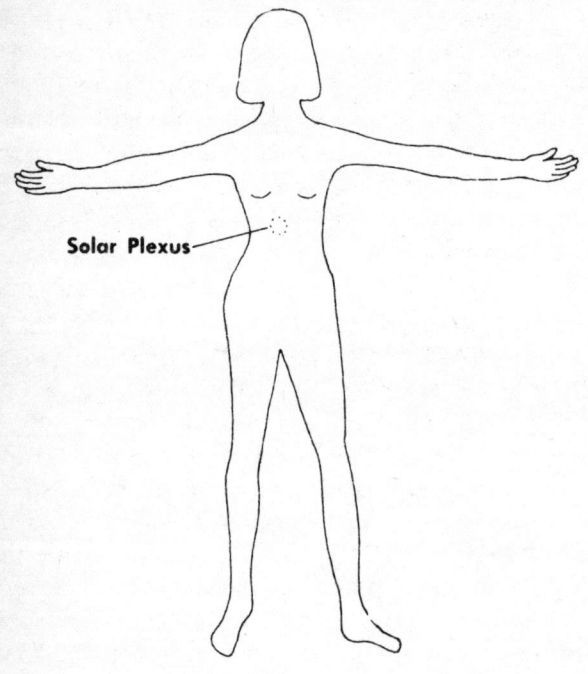

All too fanciful perhaps? If you think so, try exercises which involve breathing control alone, without the use of the imagination. Simply stretch and flex your limbs as you breathe in, feeling energy flowing up your spine. As you exhale, relax. Or take a great breath, keeping your lungs filled for as long as possible. When you have held your breath to the point of discomfort, exhale emptying your lungs completely so you cannot force out any more air. Stay empty for as long as you can, then let the air rush in. You are likely to feel exhilarated and energetic.

A final energy generator you might care to try on those occasions when you are forced to sit for long periods, particularly in a stuffy room, is the buttock tightener. Simply tense your buttocks as you inhale, and relax as you exhale. Once you can do this easily, you will find you do not actually have to move a muscle. You can do it all in your mind so onlookers do not have any idea what you are doing. This could save embarrassment.

These procedures might sound strange but such methods have been around for hundreds of years. The very fact of their survival suggests that many people have found them of value. So, try out the various exercises to be described in this chapter. Do not limit yourself by rejecting such ideas as 'outlandish' until you have experienced them. Perhaps to your surprise, you may find yourself discovering a way of effectively controlling the tension level of your body and consciously using your breathing to improve your health.

BREATHING FOR RELAXATION

It is very valuable to set aside a quiet period each day in which you relax and turn off the noise of the world for a while. Whether you make time to do so will depend on how highly you value such a quiet period compared to your other activities. It need not be a long time, even five minutes would produce discernible benefits in reducing tension and anxiety, though fifteen or twenty minutes would probably produce better results.

One way of spending this time is to practice abdominal breathing. Lie on your back, your knees bent and touching, feet about shoulder width apart on the floor. Your hands, one on top of the other, are to rest on your abdomen below your navel. Let your abdomen expand and rise as you inhale through your nose. Then allow it to sink completely as you exhale through your mouth. It is only your abdomen which moves. Your chest remains motionless. As you exhale let your body melt down into the floor, think 'relax' as you do so. Thoughts may be directed towards your body centre, just below your navel, and with each exhalation you let go more and more. Ten minutes spent in this way will be very beneficial.

Frances Halliday found this to be so. An anxious, tense person kept busy by four children and a large home, Frances was able to substitute her period of relaxed breathing for the tranquilizers which had been her crutch for over ten years. In addition to the basic abdominal breathing outlined above, she took the centering idea further. She did this in a number of ways, finding variety added enjoyment to her quiet period.

Her first centering or mental concentration exercise was to think the number 'one' as she slowly exhaled, letting this 'one' sink down and down into her abdomen below the navel. It remained there as she inhaled. On her next exhalation, Frances brought down the number 'two', placing it beside the 'one'. She continued this process until she reached 'ten' and then began again until she felt her mind descending with the numbers. When this occurred, her mind became very still and serene. She rested very peacefully for a further ten minutes.

On other occasions, Frances would descend to her body centre by mentally sliding down a rope or using a lift. In her centre she had created a sanctuary, a place where she was completely at ease. No pain or discomfort, no doubts, fears, worries or guilts could exist in this sanctuary. Everything Frances needed was there. It was hers alone, for no-one else entered her sanctuary. You may, of course, include others should you so desire. Your quiet place might be a beach, a garden, a river bank, a beautiful room, a comfortable bed, or even a warm bath. You make it what you want it to be. Probably, as you use your sanctuary it will change, developing new aspects according to your own needs.

Frances' third mind concentration technique involved breathing normally through the nose, counting 'one' as she inhaled, 'two' as she exhaled, 'three' as she inhaled again, 'four' as she exhaled again, and so on until she reached ten at which time she started again. As Frances 'counted her breaths' in this way, thoughts drifted through her mind, random thoughts which sometimes disturbed her concentration. However, she had developed a way of coping with these distractions. She thought of her mind as a room in which there were two windows, and of her random thoughts as birds. These birds would fly towards her, flying freely into her mind through one open window and out again through the other. In this way, she was able to let the thoughts go, not permitting them to stimulate further mental activity. As she did so, she returned to her counting.

These simple techniques of breathing and centering brought Frances many benefits. Each day, for twenty minutes, she 'took a holiday' from pressures, stress and bustle. She simply stopped the world and got off. By doing so, she enjoyed the tranquility of resting in a peaceful sanctuary free from anxiety provoking thoughts. Further, she proved to herself that she had considerable control over her thinking. She did not have to react to every random thought that drifted into her mind but could choose those she wished to pursue. Using the 'mind with windows' concept, Frances could simply shut the windows when a pleasant, relaxing thought entered her mind and pursue this further. Thus she could choose thoughts and feelings which promoted health and healing, a point to be elaborated in the next section.

The idea of a relaxation session every day is not confined to those who are at home, although someone in Frances' position does have the advantage of a quiet room in which to unwind. Many business people, for instance, take part of their lunchtime for a quiet time, hanging up a 'Do Not Disturb' sign on the door, taking the telephone off the hook (or arranging for their calls to be held), and stretching out on the carpet. Other people relax in their cars which they drive to a beach or park. If you really want to 'take a holiday' each day, it is only your own apathy or lack of inventiveness which will stop you. Maybe you will wait till you arrive home after work, or in the evening after dinner. When you take your quiet time is unimportant. Just give it a trial for a week or two and you will be pleasantly surprised how the feeling of relaxation it engenders stays with you for hours afterwards.

This idea of concentration upon your breathing is an important ingredient of most relaxation techniques. Basically, it involves clearing your mind of thought, focussing only upon the way you breathe. You observe consciously how you take in air, how you retain it, how you let it go. The pauses between these actions occupy your attention too, and you do all this making no effort to change your normal breathing pattern. You observe what is. It is so simple, yet so effective—turning off the endless stream of anxiety-producing thoughts which can occupy our minds so easily. Try this 'following the breath' the next time you are kept waiting, or on an occasion when you are fretful and tense. Because breathing is such a passive process requiring no deliberate effort from you, you can focus on it, letting it happen, and achieving a delightful state of deep relaxation and detachment.

Focussing on your breathing can still the jabbering voice or voices within your mind. How rarely are we internally silent? There seems always to be this never ending noise within, but you can learn to turn it off and enjoy increasingly long periods of stillness if you so desire. As you inhale, think only of your breath and be without words. Speak out the words within your mind as you exhale. With practice, the periods of inner silence can be extended, the number of words reduced. It is a marvellous feeling to experience this stillness, this quietness of mind.

Breathing and imagination go hand-in-hand to help you relax. Should your upper body feel tense and strained, try imagining you are enjoying a shower, the warm water streaming down over your head, neck, arms and shoulders. You draw the pleasant warmth into you with each inhalation and let it wash away the tension with each exhalation. Feel the shower directing warm water from the top of your spine to the bottom, and relax in its comfort.

The tripod exercise will help you 'let go' too. Sit on the edge of a straight chair with your legs planted firmly on the floor like two vertical columns. Think of your spine stretching down through the chair to the floor, forming a tripod with your two legs. As you exhale, let the tension flow down your spine into the ground.

BREATHING AND HEALING

Actually, all the various breathing techniques so far described are related to healing in one form or another. However, there are others more specifically oriented towards this end. Some, such as those outlined by Beata Jencks in her booklet *Respiration for Relaxation, Invigoration and Special Accomplishment*, really depend upon the linking of particular thoughts with the breathing pattern. We have seen examples of this approach on pages 191-93 relating to energizing and relaxation.

David Keats accepts Jencks' ideas, and uses her 'prescriptions' when he is beset by common ailments. To clear his *sinuses*, he lies in a slightly reclined position and, should it be his right nostril which is congested, with his head a little back to the left. He presses on his left nostril without closing it completely. Breathing calmly in and out, David allows air to pass through the right nostril. After several minutes, the congestion usually disappears.

Should David be discomforted by a *running nose*, he thinks 'cool and dry' as he inhales. However, if his *nose is stuffy or dry*, he concentrates on his exhalations, thinking 'warm, wide and moist' as he does so. *Sore throats* are treated by imagining moist, comfortably warm air flowing through during exhalations. David handles *coughs* by thinking 'cool, still' on inhalation and 'moist, calm, comfortable' as he exhales.

Eye problems, to which David has been subject in the past, he now handles in the following way. Exhaling gently he closes his eyes. As he inhales he feels coolness streaming gently up his nose. His next gentle exhalation relaxes the tissues around his cheekbones and above his eyes, which he allows to move under his closed lids. During inhalations he imagines air streaming in through his closed lids, thinking 'my eyes are becoming cool', and during exhalations he relaxes deeply. Where appropriate he might link thoughts to his exhalation, 'let go', or 'loose' to relieve tension, and 'dark and comfortable' to calm disturbing eye movements.

The same technique works for *aches and pains*. When

David's joints are stiff and painful, he imagines placing a drop of oil in each one, and, then, during exhalations, either actually moves the joint or imagines himself doing so. He actually feels the oil spreading throughout the hip, knee or ankle, easing movement. David's father, initially a scoffer at his son's weird notions, now uses this 'treatment' for his arthritic knee with good results. Alternatively, he may choose to think of his knee, and other joints, as composed of flexible rubber. The actual visualization used does not matter. All that matters is that you find a way of combating your pain and discomfort.

Itching, for example, certainly produces discomfort. Often it may be relieved by imagining yourself breathing through the affected skin area, keeping the thought 'cool' in your mind as you inhale and 'calm' or 'relaxed' during exhalation. David's wife, Joy, uses this technique for her *urticaria* with positive results. She also uses another of Jencks' ideas to control her attacks of nausea. She inhales 'coolness', breathing imaginatively through a hole in the small of her back. From this point she brings coolness to the inside of the upper body, and, during exhalations, relaxes the lower body. *Heartburn* may be relieved similarly. The thought is 'cool' during inhalation and 'calm' during exhalation. Alternatively, you could imagine yourself drinking milk which cools and calms the body's internal organs.

Aches and pains of all descriptions yield to either warmth or coolness. It is a matter of experimentation to find what works best for you on particular ailments. A basic technique is to imagine warmth (or coolness) in your hand which is then placed on the painful area. As you inhale, you imagine warmth (or coolness) flowing into the afflicted part, and pain streaming out and away from it during exhalation. Perhaps you might also care to imagine, during exhalation, a warm water bottle placed on the painful area, or 'see' and 'feel' a pain killing injection being administered. For *headaches*, you could imagine opening up your head at its crown during inhalations and allow coolness to stream in. As you exhale, further imagine the bony walls of the skull expanding.

Backache, a constant problem for so many people, can be

relieved through use of a warm glowing light bulb. 'See' it on the top of the head, and let it float down the spine, bringing ease and comfort. If there is a particularly painful area, first work the bulb above and below it, then imagine it on the sore spot during both inhalation and exhalation, concentrating on whichever of these brings most relief.

In a more general way, should you feel ill, sit by an open window and practice abdominal breathing for five or ten minutes. This is particularly valuable for *digestive upsets* when you feel very gassy. Alternatively you may care to imagine yourself as a bottle, your pelvis being the bottom and your mouth the top. Inhale slowly through the nose 'seeing' the bottle fill from the bottom up. When it is full, hold your breath a moment, then empty the bottle by exhaling through the mouth. This exercise has a toning up effect on the whole system.

RHYTHMIC BREATHING

Various forms of rhythmic breathing are seen as embodying healing properties. Perhaps the best known, 'the healing breath', is a cycle of inbreathing, breath holding and outbreathing performed to a count which is always in the ratio of 1:4:2. David Keats, to whom I referred earlier, practices this healing breath on his after dinner walk. He inhales for 3 strides, holds his breath for 12, and exhales for 6, repeating this procedure five times. He first began with a 2–8–4 pattern but found his lung capacity increased as he practised.

There are many other rhythmic breathing patterns, of course. David's wife tried the 1:4:2 cycle but did not feel at all comfortable with it. However, as she walks, Joy breathes in while taking 5 strides, filling her lungs as fully as possible, and then expels this air completely over the next 5 strides. This makes her feel good and has increased her lung capacity. Often she uses this 5:5 cycle when feeling lethargic and tired. She will sit and do three or four cycles of five seconds inhaling and five seconds exhaling. As she inhales, she thinks 'vitality, zest' and as she exhales 'calm, peace'.

This pattern seems to work well for Joy. She certainly thinks so. However, many experts would consider holding the breath is as important, perhaps more so, than breathing in and out. They claim, too, that it is preferable to take longer over exhaling and holding breath than over inhaling. The main thing, though, is to establish a rhythm, this being more important than the length of the breath. Practise until you get a 'feel' for the rhythm of the vibration through your whole body. When this occurs, you will find you can 'lift' yourself, clear your head, relieve aches and pains, and generally help yourself to feel much better.

In my experience, the particular rhythmic breathing pattern best designed to achieve that desirable state of affairs is this one. Firstly, establish a rhythm set by your body's pulse beat. Once you become familiar with the timing of 6 pulse beats, sit quietly breathing and counting. Then breathe in very fully for the time it takes for your pulse to beat 6 times; hold your breath for 3 beats; exhale for 6 beats; and stay empty for 3. You should get good results breathing in this way, but will enhance the effect by breathing through one nostril at a time.

Place tips of index and middle fingers of your right hand on your forehead just above the eyebrows. This enables you to pass your right thumb against the right nostril and close it, and your third and little fingers against your left nostril, and close it. To begin a cycle of single nostril rhythmic breathing, open your left nostril, exhaling completely. Close your left nostril for 3 pulse beats; open left nostril and inhale for 6 beats; close left nostril (and concentrate on centre of your forehead should you so desire) for a 3 count; open right nostril and exhale for 6 counts; close right nostril for 3 count; and so on. Though I'm using a 3:6:3:6 pattern, you may care to experiment with others, such as 4:8:4:8. The ratio of 1:2:1:2 is, however, to remain constant. This procedure sounds far more complicated when written down than it is to actually do. All that is involved is opening or closing one nostril at a time, a process which seems to be particularly effective in clearing the brain and improving mental functioning.

To engender a feeling of well-being, another variant you

could try is this. Sit on the edge of a chair with your back straight. Empty your lungs completely. Inhale through your mouth for 12 counts (pulse beats or seconds). As you breathe in for the first 4, let your stomach push out; for the next 4 let your chest rise up; and for the last 4 raise your shoulders. Hold your breathe for 4 counts, then slowly exhale through the nostrils, letting shoulders, chest and abdomen go in the reverse order. Keep lungs empty for 4 counts and begin again.

YOGIC HEALING

Much of the material on healthy breathing is derived from yoga practices. The yoga system embodies the belief that through rhythmic breathing and controlled thought, it is possible to absorb *prana* (Vital Force or Life Force) from the atmosphere and use it to heal both yourself and other people. In this latter case, you will breathe rhythmically several times until a rhythm is established, and then place your hands lightly upon the affected part of the other person's body. Continuing to breathe rhythmically, you hold the mental image that you are 'pumping' *prana* into the affected area, driving out the diseased condition. As you inhale, 'see' yourself lifting the pump handle and, as you exhale, 'see' yourself pumping the handle forcing *prana* through your hands into the other person. You are merely the machine connecting the patient to the universal supply of *prana*, a conduit which permits a free energy flow.

To vary the procedure, you may wish to stroke the patient's body with your fingertips. The basic idea is that you are bathing the other person in a flow of Vital Force which pours from your fingertips irrespective of whether you touch him or not. To increase the power of this force, you might like to concentrate your gaze and attention upon the affected part.

Should you wish to apply this procedure to heal yourself, lie flat on the floor or bed, completely relaxed, hands resting lightly on your solar plexus, and breathing rhythmically. Imagine drawing in Vital Energy with each breath, and storing it in the solar plexus. At each exhalation, will this *prana* to be distributed over every part of the body. 'See' the *prana* coming in through your lungs, being absorbed by the solar plexus, and recharging each part of the body in turn.

If you are experiencing pain, 'see' the *prana* you send healing the affected area, 'feel' the warmth of its beneficial influence as it drives out the discomfort. To speed up the process, put your hand over the painful area and, as you exhale, send a current of *prana* down your arm. Both hands may be used in this way, and as you send the Vital Force through them to the painful area, hold the image of the pump in your mind. As you pump clean, pure water (*prana*) into a pail of dirty water (the afflicted area) you will drive out the latter and replace it with the former.

According to yoga philosophy, your body has seven vital centres—the forehead, back of the head, base of the brain, solar plexus, lower part of the spine, navel region and genital region. You can revitalize your whole system by visualizing each of these centres in turn and sending a current of *prana* to it. Do this on a regular basis and you will be practicing a very effective form of preventive medicine.

Part 4
The Power of the Mind

13. Using Your Mind to Promote Good Health

MIND AND BODY

Liza Hanlon is a hypochondriac. She believes she is sick — always. One ailment follows another with monotonous regularity. Liza really suffers but she is creating her own illness by the way she chooses to think. If she is in the presence of someone who has influenza, she 'knows' she will catch that disease. Continually she worries about her state of health, mentally going over her body to check where she is feeling pain. Should she be required to 'perform' in some way, such as attending a parent-teachers night to enquire about her son's progress, or conduct a dinner party for her husband's business colleagues, she 'knows' she will be unwell on that occasion — and she is. Her problems are physical — high blood pressure, high pulse rate, muscular tension, frequent throat infections, and narrowed body cavities which produce a variety of respiratory ailments — but the cause is mental.

Mind and body are inseparable. When we are stressed emotionally, our minds full of anxiety, worry, fear, anger and jealousy, we overstimulate our adrenal glands, pouring into the body a flood of unneeded adrenalin. If such over-stimulation becomes the normal pattern of our lives, and so often it does, deleterious physical changes tend to occur similar to those experienced by Liza. That is, we can create our own illness.

However, if we can make ourselves sick through the way we think, then it would seem possible for us to improve our health by the same means. This seems rather obvious, yet people's behaviour would suggest that it is not so. The negative aspect of psychosomatic illness is widely accepted, that perhaps eighty-five per cent of the patients occupying doctors' waiting rooms are there as a result of ailments created by illness-promoting thinking. Yet, the converse, that a person can create a state of well-being through health-promoting thinking, is not a well accepted view. Perhaps this is just one more example of our human inclination to think negatively rather than positively, to fear the worst rather than expect the best. If mental states produce the physical effects noted above, this would seem very much a self-defeating policy in which we are our own worst enemies.

We do not have to be, of course. Norman Cousins, referred to in the first chapter, is living proof of the powers of a positive mental attitude. So, too, are many of Dr Carl Simonton's cancer patients. An American oncologist, Simonton practises traditional medicine, treating his patients with the conventional chemotherapy and radiation. However, in addition, he provides less traditional measures such as guided imagery and meditative visualization.

Three times a day his patients, who are usually terminal cases with no apparent hope of cure, relax deeply and visualize their illness. In these 'movies of the mind' they see their cancer, perhaps as a cauliflower or an octopus, and imagine an army of healthy white blood cells attacking it. These cells might be 'seen' as gardeners, cutting back and uprooting the cauliflower, or as frogmen cutting off the tentacles of the octopus, reducing it in size, piece by piece until it is finally destroyed. All sorts of imagery are used, the only criterion being that it is something a particular patient can use and believe in. The cancer could be a mound of dirt sucked up by defenders visualized as powerful vacuum cleaners, or a castle being destroyed by knights in shining white armour.

The basic ingredient of this approach is that the patient focuses on a positive image. Even if he cannot actually 'see' this in his mind, by just thinking about it he can strengthen his immune system and create an attitude of mind more conducive to fighting his cancer. The body has natural defences against cancer, yet it would seem that certain psychological variables interfere with these. Simonton has found, for example, that people tend to get cancer within twelve to eighteen months of a major psychological shock, such as the loss of a spouse.

He believes, though, that what really kills his cancer patients is their belief structure. That is, they believe they have an incurable disease about which they can do nothing. As soon as they are willing to accept the possibility that by mental effort they may be able to influence their physical body, many are able to create their own healing. Not all, of course. Recent reports suggest that approximately ten per cent of Simonton's patients are cured, and approximately twenty per cent definitely improved. Not impressive? Yet, these people were initially diagnosed as incurable.

Simonton stresses the importance of the body's natural defences against cancer, helping his patients to adopt a more positive attitude towards life. What he is doing is giving them the hope that through their own efforts they may be able to assist their bodies to overcome the malignant cells. It all revolves around the will to live, for, without this Simonton believes, the body will not be able to resist the disease. All of us, it would appear, have cancer. Yet, there is within us a force which keeps it in check. According to Simonton and others who think like him, this force is closely connected with a person's state of mind.

If we are able to believe that thoughts take root in our bodies as well as our minds, then it does follow that by deliberately taking more control over our thoughts we can change our bodies. It is possible to control our thinking. My previous book, *The Plus Factor*, describes some of the ways in which this might be accomplished. By taking such control, we become active participants in our own healing instead of passive victims of our disease.

We may even be able to find out why we become ill. As part of his treatment, Simonton asks his patients to look for an answer to the question: 'Why did I need my cancer in the first place?.' That is, he believes people become ill for a reason, often one they create themselves. Perhaps your pendulum might help you find an answer, or you might like to try the exercise described on pages 39-40 to tap the information you hold in your subconscious mind. Understanding what your disease is trying to tell you is often the first step in a new co-operative relationship between your mind and body, which can result in a healthier lifestyle.

Though Simonton is working with terminally ill cancer patients, his ideas have a general applicability to all of us who want to improve our health. Expressed simply, the theory is that our thoughts and our feelings create, to a great extent, our body state. To increase the possibility of good health, it behoves us to dwell more on thoughts of love, joy, peace and harmony rather than on more negative emotions. A simple prescription, but one which has not been easy to put into practice if mankind's history is any guide. However, as a personal prescription, how can we make it work?

When you take any substance which is designed to heal you, be it drug, natural remedy or food, adopt a totally positive attitude, believing confidently that it will help you. It has been suggested that up to eighty-five per cent of the efficacy of drugs and remedies generally is a function of their placebo character so our belief in a substance's healing power may do more to promote a cure than any inherent property of the substance itself.

It has been repeatedly demonstrated that belief vitally affects results produced by medications. One interesting experiment had two doctors administering the same placebo to two groups of patients. Though the substance administered was simply a milk sugar pill, one doctor suggested to his patients that it would increase their stomach acidity. It did, by an average of twelve per cent. The other doctor suggested to his patients it would decrease stomach acidity. It did, by an average of fifteen per cent. Same substance, but different beliefs about its effects.

This and similar experiments indicate that your psychological state can profoundly modify the influence a drug has upon your body. Drugs usually provide only relief of symptoms rather than producing an actual cure, but a curative effect can be created by the way you choose to think. If you believe you are taking a powerful remedy to relieve your pain, the chances are good it will have that effect even if you happen to take the wrong medication by mistake. That is, you control your body's reactions, at least to some extent, through your belief. The hypochondriac does this all the time though the control is exerted in a negative direction. Your task is to use this force positively so that you can help yourself rather than make yourself ill.

Actually, you can assume considerable control over your body by an attitude you adopt even when you know it to be false. Even if you really feel anger and fear, emotions likely to produce strain and illness, you can act as if you are happy and optimistic. You play a role, expressing positive rather than negative emotions, and it would seem that your body adjusts to this attitude despite the fact you know it to be simulated. However, the interesting thing which often happens is that we become the role we play. To become more positive, if this is what you wish, act as if you were happy and optimisitc.

In addition to changes in your mental attitude, you need to be aware of the things you say. Both inner and outer talk can be very damaging psychologically, for the things we say exert tremendous influence over our lives. Do not talk about sickness and disease. I'm sure you all know someone, or probably many someones, who do this constantly. Liza Hanlon, referred to at the beginning of this chapter, delights in telling people about her operations. This is behaviour not designed to achieve health through a positive mental attitude. If Liza is to lift herself from the state of ill-health she has created for herself, she would be better advised to think and talk about good health, for like would seem to produce like.

It has been said so often that, to a large extent, we make our lives what they are. It is generally not the events of life which make us ill, depressed and fatigued. Rather, it is our reactions to these events, and this reaction we can choose. We make our own reality by the way we choose to talk to ourselves about the events that happen to us. Whereas Liza says: 'I will get a cold' when she comes in contact with someone who sneezes all over her, another person will say: 'I never get colds.'

THE POWER OF SUGGESTION

If a person's inner and outer talk exerts such an influence on his health, it would seem a reasonable theory to hold that our well-being is largely a matter of our self-suggestion. If this is so, it behoves us to maximize the effect of suggestion so that it will work in our favour as powerfully as possible. There are several principles held to be of great importance in the use of suggestion whether it be directed toward other people or toward ourselves.

Wording suggestions positively rather than negatively is the first of these. John Sawyer, a lawyer of my acquaintance, often develops headaches. To cope with this problem, John initially sought medical advice and ascertained that there was nothing physically wrong. This is only a provisional diagnosis, of course. All the doctor can say is that the usual medical tests revealed no abnormality. Accepting this reassurance, John explored other avenues. He found auto-suggestion to be quite successful, and would always phrase his suggestion in this way. My head is becoming clear, comfortable and at ease.' He avoided any use of the word headache, for this would bring the idea of discomfort more strongly to the attention of the subconscious mind. Accordingly, suggestions like 'My headache is going' are best avoided.

Secondly, John's *suggestions are permissive* rather than authoritative. Thus, 'you *are able* to think clearly and comfortably' is used rather than 'you *will* think clearly and comfortably'. Most people respond better to the first approach than to the more dominating second approach. The same holds true of our subconscious minds which often seem to resist commands. In your own use of suggestion, you could try both types, perhaps using a permissive suggestion first and, should that not be successful, become more authoritative.

Repetition, the third principle, is often seen as the key to effective suggestion. I am in some doubt about this myself. Repeating a suggestion three or four times on numerous occasions does seem to work well for many people. Yet John often gets excellent results by a single statement. A particular form of suggestion, stated in question form once only, which he sometimes uses is, 'What do I have to do for my head to become clear and comfortable?.' This is positive and permissive. It is really asking the subconscious mind to come up with an answer, and this it usually does without further repetition being necessary. Again, you will need to discover what works best for you.

Once John makes his suggestion, he allows time for his subconscious mind to accept the suggestion. That is, he does not say, 'My head is clear and comfortable' for that would seem ridiculous in the face of a pounding headache. Instead he phrases it this way: 'My head is becoming increasingly clear and increasingly comfortable and will soon be completely at ease.'

Suggestions may take the form of silent thoughts or words spoken aloud. They can be directed at I: 'I will feel at ease' or at you: 'You will feel at ease.' Use which you feel most comfortable with or a mixture if you so desire, linking the verbal suggestion with a visual image. Study a book of anatomy, for example, so that when you imagine a particular organ you know what it looks like in its healthy state. A sore throat, red and inflamed, could be treated with the verbal suggestion: 'My throat is pink and moist' together with an image of the throat looking this way and feeling normal.

Don't overdo the suggestions. Concentrate on one, or at most, two things at a time. You can be quite specific about your goal, setting up an image of, for example, the healthy throat, as a goal for the subconscious mind toward which the suggestion is directed. Conversely, you might like to use a more general statement such as that proposed by Emile Coué earlier this century: 'Every day in every way I am getting better and better.' This non-specific approach permits the sub-conscious mind to focus on whatever seems important at the time. Note, too, the use of 'am'. You assume the suggestion will work. Avoid the word 'try' which implies doubt.

Galen, one of the most famous of early physicians, said: 'When the imagination of a sick man has been struck with an idea of a remedy, which is in itself without efficacy, it becomes endowed with beneficent power.' This is what occurs when we suggest healing to ourselves and, in this sense, suggestion is really just another name for placebo. Placebos given for pain relief apparently release a natural pain killing substance in the brain termed endorphins. Jogging and meditation are also claimed as methods through which endorphins can be released. Possibly positive suggestion might do likewise, thus strengthening the body's own healing powers.

Certainly, it can promote curative effects quite rapidly. Professor Hans Eysenck of London's Maudsley Hospital performed an interesting experiment attesting to this. Two groups of children were involved, one receiving orthodox medical treatment for warts, the other receiving suggestion. Using a large sheet of paper, this latter group drew pictures of a child's hand with warts on it. Around these warts, the children drew circles. Each day the size of the warts in the drawing was reduced until they finally disappeared, the hand being drawn in an unblemished state. The results of the experiment indicated that this treatment was far more effective in 'curing' the children's warts than the orthodox medical treatment.

Perhaps you may care to use the pendulum in association with your positive suggestion, firstly to select from among possible wordings and secondly, to get some indication of success. You can, that is, ask your pendulum whether the suggestion you have used has been accepted. If the answer you receive is negative, you can question further to find how you might make your suggestions more effective.

USING SELF-HYPNOSIS TO ENHANCE THE POWER OF SUGGESTION

One way of doing so is to use self-hypnosis. The hypnotized person is not unconscious or asleep. He knows what he is saying and doing, yet usually he does not wish to speak or move because he feels delightfully peaceful. If he is in only a light trance, his sensations are little different from those he experiences when he relaxes, though, should he enter into a deep trance, he will be aware of a difference in his state.

Using Your Mind to Promote Good Health

All of us have within us a certain capacity of drift into a trance state. We do it regularly, possibly every day, entering the state spontaneously when we daydream, concentrate fully upon a book, or become deeply involved in a film. These episodes are not labelled hypnosis but the state is the same.

Many sportsmen and women spontaneously induce self-hypnosis, particularly when the activity in which they are engaged is rhythmical in nature. Cycling, swimming, rowing and distance running are examples which spring readily to mind. Religious ceremonies with their ritual music exercise a strong hypnotic influence as do the flashing lights and bass beat music of discos. Car drivers, much to their cost, have been known to enter trance states as their attention becomes fixed on the white lines of the road or the windscreen wipers as they move back and forth. Concentration of attention induces the trance.

Because hypnosis is such a common, naturally occurring state, you need have no worries about using it to enhance the power of your self-suggestions and so improve your health. The value of using it is that it increases your suggestibility, making you more responsive to the words and images you feed into your mind. Suggestion under hypnosis works well if you really want to act in the way stated. However, if you hope you can force yourself to do things you really do not want to do, you are doomed to disappointment. Your suggestions must be acceptable to you or you will simply reject them. Depth of trance, despite much literature to the contrary, is not the main thing. It is your eagerness to accept the suggestion that determines the success or otherwise of the approach. You use self-hypnosis to help you achieve the things you want to achieve.

To learn hypnosis, have a physician or therapist teach you. That is the advice most commonly given and it is sound enough. However, it is a straightforward procedure, one you can learn alone. After all, no one taught you to daydream, and self-hypnosis has been described as guided day-dreaming. One approach is to follow this sequence:
1. Seated comfortably, take a few deep breaths, thinking 'let

go' as you exhale. Focus your eyes on a spot on the ceiling, a picture on the wall, a flickering candle flame or any other object which can claim your full attention.
2. As you 'let go', concentrate exclusively upon your spot, giving yourself suggestions of eye heaviness and of eye closure. If your eyes do not close within a minute or two because of their heaviness and tiredness, deliberately shut them. Avoid straining or making your eyes feel uncomfortable.
3. Relax your muscles, starting at the feet and working up to the forehead. Either send breaths to the body or tense and relax each muscle in turn.
4. Imagine you are descending stairs or an escalator, or are going down in a lift. Count the floors or the steps, drifting deeper with each one.
5. Enter a sanctuary, or secret room in your mind where you are completely at peace, free of worry, stress and problems. Be quiet and still.
6. Give yourself suggestions verbally and visually.
7. Tell yourself you will drift into a relaxed trance state more deeply and more quickly next time.
8. Return to the 'surface' by counting to ten, drawing in energy with each breath so that when you reach ten you are alert, rested and feeling very good.

This approach is fairly typical but, if you feel it is somewhat cumbersome, I would not worry unduly. It is not really necessary to go through all those steps because, whether or not you drift into a suggestible trance state, is purely a function of the extent to which you allow yourself to 'let go'. For many people, all they need to do is close their eyes, take a deep breath or two to relax, and they are there. Others simply sit comfortably and imagine themselves in a pleasant place, 'turning off' the real world as they do. However, as a beginner, the security of a longer, more leisurely approach might be initially helpful.

A rather pleasant method you might like to explore involves mentally going through the colours of the rainbow, linking each one to a particular sensation. After relaxing yourself with several deep slow breaths, which is probably the best way to begin, think of the colour red. Perhaps you have an image of a bright *red* fire engine as you do so. As you think of *orange* you may imagine yourself sucking the juice from an actual orange. *Yellow,* the next colour, could be linked to a wattle tree and the smell associated with it. *Green* might mean a place of peace, a tranquil river bank perhaps. The *blue* sky may be the next image, blending into the *indigo* of twilight. *Violet,* the final colour could, for you, be the flower, violet.

However you go about hypnotizing yourself, the essential element is that you turn off the real world and go into a world of the mind which you create for yourself. To do this, you do not have to follow set rules such as fixing your eyes on an object, or thinking of particular images. Try the various ways suggested in this section and some of the breathing exercises outlined earlier. Should you fall asleep, do not worry. You will awaken as you would from a normal sleep. Actually falling asleep after you have dropped an important suggestion into your mind is quite helpful, for the sub-conscious mind will work on it as you sleep.

Personally, I find my patients like best a self-hypnosis technique involving only two steps. Firstly, they take five deep breaths, with each exhalation letting go a little bit more so that, by the end of the five, their muscles have relaxed. They then go away to some place in their mind where they feel at peace. This sanctuary may range from a beach or forest to a bed or a warm bath. Wherever it is, they often erect a screen, sometimes large like that at a drive-in theatre, sometimes small about the size of a television set. On this screen they see themselves as they want to be, free of illness and pain, moving easily, full of energy and the joy of living. To enhance the picture, should you want to use this method, you might care to surround the image of yourself with white or golden light representing energy, healing and protection.

One way of using this screen is to first project an image of yourself as you are, with your ailment. To the left of this image place another one in which you see yourself being treated in some way. Perhaps soothing ointments are being applied, or your spine is being manipulated, or your limbs are being massaged. Whatever the form of treatment, you see it healing you. You then place a third image further left, this one showing yourself in perfect health. Alternatively you may want only to use an image of health so you implant this firmly in the mind.

Self-hypnosis is a tool, one which will help you enhance the effectiveness of your suggestions. It is also one to use if you suffer from *insomnia*. As soon as you settle into bed, induce a state of self-hypnosis. One suitable method is to hear the 'sound of calm', whatever that might be for you, each time to exhale, letting each breath carry you deeper and deeper. Another is to imagine a blackboard on which you write numbers. As you wipe off each number you let go a little more until you reach a previously decided point, say thirty. When you wipe off the number thirty you let go completely.

As you rest in the dreamy trance state you can suggest something like: 'Very soon I will drift into a deep, sound sleep which will continue undisturbed until the time I wish to awaken in the morning. (Visualize a clock face showing your awakening time at this point). I will then get up feeling very refreshed and looking forward to the new day.' You may care to put this suggestion more indirectly: 'What do I have to do to drift into a deep, sound sleep?' Once you have put the suggestion into your mind, turn your thoughts from sleep. Think of this as a valuable time to practise relaxation or correct breathing. As you do, the chances are quite good you will slip naturally into sleep.

THE PROBLEMS OF STRESS

Insomnia is part of a wider problem, that of emotional tension. The prevalence of emotional stress is seen, by many, as a result of the competitive ethic that is instilled into us from an early age. Co-operation, though given much lip-service, usually yields to the fierce desire to do something better than someone else. Behaviour of this sort puts considerable strain upon us for there are always new pressures, new demands to perform better than our peers.

Together with this training in competitiveness goes an injunction on the free expression of emotion. This is aimed primarily at males who are expected to present a relatively unemotional exterior, marked by the stiff upper lip. This emotional restraint is reflected in our posture. As Wilhelm Reich has pointed out, we create a body armour for ourselves, tensing abdominal muscles, clenching our jaws, and generally imposing a certain rigidity upon ourselves. Each of us tends to create this armour for self-defence, to help us handle emotionally laden situations, but it becomes our prison, blocking the expression of emotion and even restricting our movements.

Time, too, can be an enemy, one which increases the stress of our environment. We can allow ourselves to become locked in a constant battle with time, struggling to meet deadlines, trying to do things as fast as possible, often without realizing these same things are not really worth doing anyway. Without stopping to think about the value of what we do, we pile one task on top of another, increasing the load, increasing the tension.

A certain level of tension is, of course, necessary if we are to function effectively. A life without stress would be very dull indeed, for we require the occasional stimulus of fear and anxiety to keep us alert. However, stress becomes a problem, a harmful influence when it is unrelieved. That is, for many of us, a high state of tension is a permanent part of our lives. Our bodies are constantly in a state of readiness to fight or flee and we are locked into a health-damaging cycle. We try hard to relax, and the harder we try, the more tense we become. Relaxation is not something that comes with effort. It is something we have to let happen.

You can ascertain quite easily whether you exist in this stressed state. Do you wake in the morning feeling tired and depressed? Is your resting pulse rate during the day usually over seventy? Do you suffer from stiff necks, headaches, facial wrinkles and worry lines? If so, you are likely to be over-stressed.

Tranquilizers, the usual 'remedy' for such a state, are not the answer. We need to learn how to relax. Perhaps the form of relaxation you choose is physical. If, after exposure to stress, you take some form of vigorous activity you are likely to work off most of your tension. Swimming, jogging, brisk walking and cycling are all excellent activities to achieve this end. As Dr Donald Norfolk puts it in the *Habits of Health*: 'Exercise . . . is the perfect antidote for stress: regular relaxation the ideal prophylactic.' So, one way to reduce your stress level is to exercise when you feel tense and take brief relaxation periods during the day to prevent too much tension developing.

The point about stress we must keep constantly in mind is that it is not something out there in the world waiting to damage us. It comes from within. We create our own stress by our internal thought processes, by the way we choose to view life. If you are over-stressed it is because you have elected to react to people and things in a way that fills you with tension and anxiety.

Once you realize you are responsible for your stress, you can do something about it. However, if you believe you are a 'born worrier', or a 'tense personality', or that you inherited your tension tendencies, you haven't a chance of improving matters. Holding a view that your behaviour and emotional state was determined at birth, you will not make any effort to find ways of controlling your worrying thoughts, of curbing your impatience with others, of not imposing perfectionistic standards upon yourself and those around you, of avoiding comparing yourself unfavourably with others, and of slowing down so you no longer hurry everything you do.

Stress, if it be your constant companion, can make you ill, primarily through reducing your resistance to infection. According to Hans Selye, acknowledged as the world's leading authority on stress-linked disease, there are three phases involved. Initially, the body reacts to fear or frustration with its chemical weapons, releasing additional adrenalin, among other things, into the bloodstream. Thus the body is readied for action. Secondly, even after the threat retreats, the body maintains its excess energy level, though this is no longer needed. Finally, should the reactions to threat last too long, biological exhaustion occurs and body organs suffer damage.

As mentioned earlier, the answer to this problem does not really lie in attaining a state of perfect serenity. Rather, each of us might try to find our own optimum level of functioning. We need to be able to identify the level of arousal at which we feel best. If we feel anxious, tense, stressed, we need to relax, to reduce our arousal level. Conversely, should we feel sluggish, lethargic and indifferent, we need to realize we are operating at too low an arousal level and that we require additional stimulation. Perhaps we engage in risk-taking activities at such times, or become more physically active, doing things we really enjoy.

Tension, then, is not bad in itself. It keys us up for important events. Most successful entertainers, sportsmen and women, and public speakers feel 'butterflies' in the stomach before they perform. It is nature's way of getting us ready for a big effort. It is only when the tension becomes too great, too constant, that we need to do something about it, for at this point it can interfere with our health.

THE RELIEF OF STRESS

Emotional stress causes physical tensions, and physical rigidity causes emotional strain. Relieve one and you relieve the other. We have mentioned exercise and breathing as ways of achieving this. There are many others of course, some mentioned in previous chapters, some now to be outlined.

There are a variety of ways you can use a period of repose which you set aside each day. I have commented on this idea before but repeat it here because many people find it the best single method of introducing more tranquillity into their lives. Simply turning off the world for ten, fifteen, twenty or thirty minutes each day is a soothing experience. You can take this period as one long session, or several short sessions during the day.

Once you decide to try out this idea, there are a number of things you can do. Perhaps you may wish to sit quietly and *meditate*. The simpler your technique the better, for the only essential element is quietness of mind, a clearing away of extraneous internal babble. A *mantra* is one way of achieving this. By concentration on the repetition of a sound, you give your mind a focus. As your mind strays away, you bring it quietly back to concentrate on your sound, which can be anything you choose, any word or words which give you pleasure. 'Love', 'Peace', 'Flower', 'Calm' are all popular choices, as is the yogic 'Om'. Your focus does not, however, need to be a sound. You can concentrate on a vase, a flower, a light, a candle flame, or anything else you wish.

Alternatively, instead of focussing your mind on a single point, you may prefer to *open the windows of your mind* and watch the thoughts as they flow through. Just let them come and go without making any effort to hold on to them.

Though meditation is usually considered as a sitting procedure, some people prefer action meditation in which, as they jog, or swim, or walk, they focus on their body's action. All other thoughts are let go and all that matters is the actual movement of the moment. Such a meditation achieves the dual purpose of syphoning off stress through exercise, and focussing the mind. It is well worth trying, too, as you go through your daily routine. Really concentrate on making the beds, washing dishes, and mowing lawns. Dreary, boring tasks? Only if you make them so. Feel textures, smell odours (if pleasant), see colours and hear sounds. Use your senses and be intensely aware. Live intensely in the present which is, in itself, a fascinating meditation.

Brian Martin provides an illustration of another way of using the quiet period. Lying on the floor, Brian stretches and yawns, then adopts the 'corpse' posture which is described on page 188. Mentally he ranges over his whole body, letting go tensions. He concentrates particularly on the jaw, tongue, eyes, forehead and hands, tensing and relaxing them in turn. Brian then focusses on his breathing which becomes slow, deep and rhythmical. He suggests his body is becoming heavy and warm, sinking down into the carpet as all tension melts away. Fantasy trips come next as Brian mentally revisits happy experiences of his past and projects forward to happy events of the future.

Finally, he suggests he will feel calm, relaxed and peaceful for the rest of the day. Brian Martin does not have ulcers, high blood pressure or tension headaches. Before he embarked on this daily routine he had all three. Perhaps his quiet time procedure is not the only reason for his improvement but Brian certainly believes it to be so.

Perhaps you may prefer to use your 'time-out' period for a catnap. Why not? A nap during the day prevents tension and fatigue accumulating, particularly if it is taken around the middle of the day. Such a break provides relief from stress and mental strain. Perhaps the siesta, so beloved of Europeans, South Americans and others, should have wider currency in our own society. Certainly, many people would seem to live their lives more productively on relatively few hours sleep at night, say four or five, and the occasional catnap during the day. Again, it is a matter of personal experiment to find the patterns which work best for you.

Sometimes when we realize our need to relax, to let go negative emotions, we just feel too fatigued or ill to bother. Yet, at times like these a session of deliberate relaxation can be of immense benefit. Keep a relaxation tape in reserve for such moments. Either record your own voice or that of a friend taking you through a series of relaxation suggestions. In this way you can simply flop, turn on the recorder, and let the tape do the work. You can also ask, as the tape does its work and eases you into peacefulness, 'What do I have to do to improve my health?.' Hopefully you'll then find fewer occasions on which you are so fatigued that you need the tape.

Our minds play a great part in our release from stress. As pointed out in Chapter 12, the imagination is a powerful calming agent. Perhaps, as you physically relax, you would like to imagine yourself standing on a ledge overlooking a pool. You pick up a large rock and drop it into the water, watching it disappear from view. The ripples spread out over the surface of the pool. You watch the water gradually becoming still again as the ripples die away and your mind becomes as still and untouched as the water.

Or you might like to engage in mental 'doodling'. Draw a

circle, clockwise, and place a dot in the centre (⊙). Do this over and over again, or draw a series of these circles smoothly and rhythmically. Then try an equilateral triangle (△), beginning at the bottom right hand corner, moving to the apex, down to the left hand corner of the base, and back to the starting point. You can keep going over the same triangle or do a number side by side. A cross (+) is another soothing 'doodle'. Start at the bottom and go to the top, then draw the crosspiece left to right.

Try separating from your body. As you lie or sit comfortably, pay attention to everything which is going on in your body. Do not analyse, simply observe and report out loud what you feel: 'Ache in the left hip', 'itch in the big toe', 'tightness in the left calf'. Notice it is not *'my* left hip' but *'the* left hip'. You are separating, distancing yourself from your body, a process which results in quietness of mind and body. This is a procedure well worth using if you are troubled by *insomnia*.

So, too, is visualizing a blank screen in your mind. Concentrate on keeping your mind free of thoughts and images, except for the screen. Each time you stray, bring your mind back to the screen and its blankness, its nothingness. Flow with such interruptions, accepting them, letting them go, and then returning to your screen. If the screen is not appealing try the same approach with a velvety black curtain.

CONTROLLING PAIN

Simply creating a quiet time for relaxation will provide some relief from pain you might be feeling. Depending on how we use our minds, we can increase or decrease pain. Should we choose to focus excessively upon our pain, our minds act as amplifiers, increasing its severity. If we are also tense or anxious, our pain will seem much greater. However, should we distract our minds, giving them something to concentrate upon other than the pain, and should we relax, letting go our tension and anxiety, we can dampen its effect. Use of the quiet period to perform some of the mental healing exercises already described will help you achieve this dampening effect.

Pain is a complex experience having both primary and

secondary components. Ron Hoddle badly twisted his knee while playing tennis. It hurt. This is Ron's primary pain. However, in addition, Ron worried about his injury. As a shopkeeper, he had to move around a lot, and there was no one who could take over for him. Thus he became increasingly anxious about how he would be able to cope. This anxiety is the secondary component of Ron's pain, the 'amplifier' which made his pain considerably greater than it need have been. His anxiety created a tension in his body which interfered with blood flow, thus reducing the supply of nutrients to the damaged area and also reducing the speed with which waste products were removed. It also *stimulated his nerve endings to transmit pain messages more strongly.*

Fortunately, a friend of Ron's, Andy, an ambulance driver told him about a pain combating technique he had used successfully with many accident victims. He suggested that Ron look upon his pain as a signal that something was wrong and needed fixing. Ron knew something was wrong all right. He could hardly walk and when he put any weight on the knee he almost screamed with agony. However, when he rested it, using alternate hot and cold fomentations, it became much easier. In addition, his medically prescribed pain killers made it possible for him to do the essential things which he felt he had to do. These he used sparingly, for emergencies only. Also, he used crutches which enabled him to move about without putting weight on his injury.

Andy pointed out that the pain signal had been noted and something done about it. The injury was being treated, and would, in time, heal. Ron could assist that healing by letting go the 'amplifier' of anxiety. One way of doing so was to close his eyes and imagine his pain as a force outside himself. Andy suggested Ron think of this outside stimulus as a telephone ringing. But this was a call Ron had no need to answer for he already knew who was calling—his pain. He had already done all he could to cope with this pain so he could let the telephone keep on ringing. This imagery helped Ron relax, and by so doing, diminish his pain. Imagery and relaxation go hand in hand, and they are powerful weapons in the control of pain.

Pain, too, has past and future components as well as those which exist in the present. The immediate pain of an injury is only one third of the total experience, but it is increased by the memory of past pain and the fear of continuing future suffering. Again it is the mind which creates this 'amplifying' effect, and by focussing your mind away from your pain, by refusing to allow thoughts of past problems and future fears to remain in your mind, you exert the control which will reduce your suffering.

One such control device is to imagine you have, in your head, a long row of electric light switches. Each of these is connected to a different part of the body and above each is a small electric light bulb. These may all be the same colour or you may like to vary colours according to the parts of the body involved. If Ron chose to work with this image, he would turn off the pain in his knee by turning off the switch and seeing the light go out. A mental 'trick'? Yes, but it is one that can reduce pain very considerably.

Colours can be used in another pain-reducing image. Think of one part of your body which is healthy. What colour do you see? Think of an injured, painful area? What colour is it? Then 'see' the colour of the injury, often a dirty, muddy colour gradually changing to the colour of health. As it does so, the pain usually lessens and the feeling of healing increases. So much of our pain is in our minds that mental manipulations of this type can offer a most effective form of control.

USING THE MIND TO CONTROL WEIGHT

Mental manipulations can also be helpful in our battle against excess weight. Perhaps the key element here is mentally 'seeing' yourself as you want to be. Visualize yourself standing on a set of scales with those scales showing the weight you want to be. 'See' yourself looking the way you want to look when you are that weight. By visualizing yourself exactly as you want to be, you are giving your subconscious mind a target, and usually it will do what is necessary to get you there. To strengthen your imagery, get out photographs of yourself when you were the weight you now wish to be. If you have clothes into which you no longer fit, get them out too, hanging them in plain sight. All this helps create the desired self-image which, implanted firmly in your mind, exerts considerable control over your eating habits.

These eating habits can be visualized, too. 'See' yourself eating small meals of low calorie, healthy foods leaving at least one bite on the plate. Visualize yourself rejecting rich, unhealthy high calorie foods, and refusing to nibble and pick while preparing food. In short, 'see' yourself as you want to be.

Use positive thinking. If you have ever managed to reduce your food intake for a single day, you can lose weight. Take one day at a time, and eat less than normal on that day. Start fresh next day, for anyone can reduce their food intake for such a short time. Do not look ahead. Of course, you will have the occasional lapses but a new day is coming up tomorrow and you can make it a good one as far as eating less food is concerned. Soon you will link a succession of these good days together and the weight starts melting away.

There is an old saying: 'It's all in the mind.' Well, perhaps not everything is mental but certainly much of our illness stems from this cause. This chapter has outlined ways in which you can reverse this process, using your mind to improve your health. As you do so, you will become increasingly aware of the immense power you have within you to take more control over your own life. It is a marvellous feeling.

14. The Healing of Faith

ORTHODOX MEDICINE— FROM FAITH TO TECHNOLOGY

Faith has been defined by Norman Shealy, the American neurosurgeon, as 'a lack of resistance to that which one hopes to receive'. Some of us do not permit faith to work for us because our scepticism establishes a resistance which faith cannot breach. We do not allow ourselves to accept the assurance of things hoped for, the conviction that things not yet visible will eventuate. A great pity, really, for trust that someone or something is working on your behalf to heal you is possibly the greatest aid to recovery from illness. What you put your trust in is often the key element in your cure whether this be a god, a spiritual healer, a doctor, or a medicine man.

In a very real sense, medicine is now, as it has always been, faith healing. This faith, according to Shealy, stems from the patient's belief that his physician really cares about him as a fellow human being, rather than seeing him as just another case. More than this, the patient senses his doctor's empathy and love. Love is vital, for there appears to be a virtually unanimous belief on the part of healers throughout the ages that healing comes from the power of love. For some this love stems from a god, for others, it is a universal love-energy, and for yet others it is something found in fellow human beings. The person who treats us warmly and with empathy, showing an understanding and sensitivity for our suffering, is usually able to heal us because we believe in him. We have faith.

Have our modern doctors cut themselves off from this source

of healing power? Shealy, among many others, believes so. In his book, *Occult Medicine*, he has pointed out that when the modern American physician abandoned his confidence-instilling 'bedside' manner, he provoked a strong reaction. The American public began complaining of the loss of the old-fashioned family doctor who, while lacking the technology of the clinic, cared for his patients in a personal way. Far more patients are now seeking treatment from practitioners of non-orthodox medicine simply because orthodox medicine is no longer able to provide what they need. Perhaps the most common characteristic of these unorthodox healers is that they regard the patient as a total human being, not as an 'illness' or a 'case'. Through his 'bedside' manner, with its warmth, love and sincerity, the old-fashioned doctor was able to mobilize the patient's expectancy of a cure. By relinquishing this approach, the modern doctor has given up his greatest healing weapon.

What has replaced it? A technological approach to *disease* care now prevails, in which it is seen as appropriate for the doctor to keep patients at arm's length. Throughout the ages, closeness, laying-on of hands, and warmth, have all proven their value in the healing process, yet modern medicine is giving up this personal touch in favour of a detached, objective scientific mode of treatment that is not meeting patients' human needs. Technology is brought to bear on the offending organ without concern for the person to whom it belongs. A human being is more than a collection of parts which may or may not be functioning well. The occasional doctor still realizes this but increasing numbers, trained in the mechanistic techniques of a technological society, behave towards their patients more as if they were machines rather than fellow human beings.

The medical profession would possibly argue that it is necessary to adopt such an approach for, if they empathized with their patients, sharing their suffering and pain, they would be rendered incapable of practising their profession. Only by remaining detached and objective are they able to perform their healing function. Perhaps this view has merit, but it does not seem to impede the work of the unorthodox practitioners whom patients are seeking out with increasing frequency. The key point is that of faith. If a doctor, while remaining remote and detached, can maintain his patient's faith that he can heal him, then he has achieved a very workable compromise. However, this is a compromise which relatively few medical practitioners seem able to achieve.

If most illness were organic in nature, perhaps the problem outlined above would not be a serious one. However, when we realize that approximately eighty-five per cent of the diseases a doctor sees are psychosomatic in origin, it is clear that most patients do not need to be treated with technology but with something as non-physical as the complaint itself. A non-physical factor such as faith must obviously be of great importance in the treatment of psychosomatic illness for, as has been already pointed out, if a mind can produce illness it can also produce health and healing. To do so, a change of attitude on the part of the sufferer is required and faith, a positive attitude, has often proven to be the catalyst which effects this change.

Psychosomatic illness does seem to be the weak point of orthodox medicine. Medical students are rarely taught how to deal with such disorders, possibly because the profession as a whole is uncertain how the problem should be handled. Drugs, the most commonly used treatment, are really no answer. Sedatives, narcotics and tranquilizers often mask the problem, leaving it untouched and adding the possibility that the patient may develop a drug addiction as well. The peculiar situation exists, then, that the most common medical problem in the community is one which traditional medicine is ill-equipped to handle. In fact, the movement away from the more personalized medicine of the past to the scientifically detached technological approach of the present seems to have eroded the doctor's ability to help people suffering from psychosomatic disorders.

Because of this void left by modern medicine, increasing numbers of patients are seeking help from practitioners of unorthodox medicine. Whether their natural food cures, their homoeopathic, Bach and Schuessler remedies, their water treatments, their acupressure and acupuncture treatments, and their spinal manipulations are any more effective than the drugs and surgery of orthodox medicine can only be determined by personal experience. However, because unorthodox practitioners care for the whole person they seem successful in mobilizing the faith of the people they treat. The many cures they achieve, then, with patients suffering psychosomatic illnesses, may be more a function of this faith than the particular methods they use. We all appear to need faith in something, a fact well illustrated by the now famous example of the Krebiozen experiment.

A patient with a far advanced cancer sought entry to a study of a new anti-cancer drug named Krebiozen. Initally, his request was refused because his case was so bad that he was felt to be an inappropriate subject to use in the experiment. As he had no hope of recovery from his illness, his use of the new drug would be a waste of time. However, so insistent was he, that he was finally given the medication and included in the study. Having read about the miraculous powers claimed for Krebiozen, the patient had developed a great faith in its ability to cure him. Accordingly, he was not surprised when his tumour masses 'melted like snowflakes on a hot stove'. His doctors, however, certainly were surprised, for this patient, who previously required an oxygen mask to breathe, became fully active, left hospital and even flew his plane at an altitude of 4000 metres with no ill effects.

After some time, reports appeared in the press that Krebiozen had not lived up to expectations, the experiment revealing that it was ineffective as a cancer cure. The patient's tumour masses returned and he again became hospitalized and confined to bed. Impressed by the patient's previous positive reaction to an apparently ineffective drug, the physician in charge of his case restored his faith by telling him the Krebiozen apparently deteriorated upon standing. This was the reason for the poor results which were quoted in the press. To overcome this problem, he would be given a double strength dose. The injection was actually water. Despite this, the same amazing recovery took place. The apparently terminal cancer remitted and the patient resumed his normal life. Unfortunately, a little later an official announcement emanating from the American

Medical Association stated that Krebiozen was of no value in the treatment of cancer. Within a few days the patient was dead.

We all have faith in something. This patient had faith in a 'miracle' cure. Others have faith in a benign god, an aspect to be discussed in the next section. Unfortunately, some of us have faith in failure, sickness, and misfortune. When we are told to have faith we need to realize we already have faith. The question we must ask ourselves is whether our faith is constructive, improving our health, or negative, creating illness and suffering. We also need to maintain our positive faith in the face of efforts, often well meaning, which actually exert a negative effect upon us. This is illustrated beautifully in the testimony of a satisfied patient giving evidence to a nineteenth-century French inquiry into faith healing:

> If it is an illusion to which I owe the health I believe I enjoy, I humbly entreat the experts who see so clearly, not to destroy it; that they may enlighten the Universe, that they leave me with my error, and that they permit my simplicity, my frailty, and my ignorance to make use of an invisible agent which does not exist but which cures me.

This is the nub of the matter. If, through your faith in a god, a doctor, a remedy, a food, or a vitamin pill, you improve your health, ignore statements which tell you these things are useless. Strengthen your faith, for by so doing you are co-operating with a tremendously powerful healing force.

RELIGIOUS FAITH

It is now fashionable to belittle religion yet, again, the sceptic may be blocking himself off from a beneficial influence which the more credulous enjoy. By holding fast to faith in a god, or any other healing power, a person has created for himself a constant source of support. It really does not matter, in this context, whether a god actually does or does not exist. It is a person's belief which is all important because it is this belief that governs his behaviour. He behaves 'as if' a god exists, or 'as if' the shrine at Lourdes will heal him. If we believe a god exists, then for us, he, she or it does exist.

Evelyn Flowers possessed such a belief. A regular church attender, she had enjoyed good health for most of her life, a circumstance she attributed to her piety. Then she became ill, running a high fever, aching all over, perspiring profusely and breaking out in a violent skin eruption. Drugs provided little relief, blood tests showed no abnormality and Evelyn prayed for healing. No healing came. Her illness was long and protracted and her faith in the power of prayer disappeared. Her god had failed her.

Or had he? In her book *The Healing Light*, Christian writer Agnes Sanford has argued that it is not a lack in God if our prayers fail but a natural and understandable lack in ourselves. If our initial attempts at healing ourselves through prayer are unproductive, it is only because we have not found the appropriate way of contacting God. She suggests we adopt an experimental attitude to our prayers until we find the most effective way of tapping God's power.

Evelyn learnt about Sanford's idea from a neighbour who dropped in to comfort her. Despite her bitterness over the previously unsuccessful efforts to ask God's help, she decided to try again. In fact, she was in an ideal situation to do so for Sanford suggests that our first prayer-experiments should involve an object that is simple and personal, such as the healing of our bodies. Praying for healing is a natural and instinctive action expressing a desire for harmony with God. Evelyn, then, went ahead, prayed, and observed the results to judge whether her prayers had been effective. If the particular approach she adopted failed, as had her first attempt, she would seek a better adjustment with God and try again until she found an approach that worked.

In Evelyn's case this was not necessary. As she heard more about Sanford's ideas from her neighbour, she realized that her first attempt at enlisting God's healing help consisted entirely of pleading, of asking. This time she used her prayer of faith which involves:

1. Knowing what the god has promised in the religious writing.

2. Believing that you receive these promises with no doubt in your head.

According to this view, if prayer is to be answered, we have to believe our prayer is being answered, that we are already receiving that for which we have asked. We need to think of it as an accomplished fact, and to give thanks for the healing that is taking place within us.

Evelyn, then, prayed for healing and gave thanks to her god before anything actually happened. This is true faith, for she gave thanks for an answer before the answer was seen. She was grateful for her god's healing even though such healing was not immediately apparent. The prayer of faith, then, means thanking your god and continuing to thank, believing the prayer is being answered. It also means that you have what you accept.

This is true whether your god is the Christian one of the Bible or any other god in whom you believe. Agnes Sanford, world famous for her exposition of healing through religious faith, works within the Christian concept and, because I am using her approach as an example of the prayer of faith, it may appear as if I advocate this framework only. This is not so, for it is the very existence of belief in a powerful, beneficent being or force which is the key to healing, not the particular god who is invoked. As long as you can contact your god in such a way that you achieve healing, it seems pointless to argue theology.

Healing energy is within us and in the world around us. To receive more of it, we ask for it. Obviously, we can only do so if we believe there is something outside ourselves which can answer this request and help nature to heal our injury. So the prayer of faith involves:

1. Making yourself comfortable and relaxing, the body and mind quiet and still;
2. Reminding yourself of the reality of the life outside of you, labelled god or universal force;
3. Asking that life to come in and heal you;
4. Making a picture in your mind of your body well, as you want it to be;

5. Giving thanks for the healing you are receiving.

This idea appears in so many cultures that perhaps it approaches the status of a universal truth. By making a picture in our minds of the basic good health we expect, and by then accepting through faith that it will be so, we seem to release great healing power. This can be imagined as a kind of light, shining, burning, glowing and flowing through the body, concentrated on the diseased part.

Evelyn's experiment proved successful, for her health did improve. Not suddenly, for it is the rare case when instant cures are affected, but progressively her body became stronger and the effects of her illness receded. She had sought help from her god by contacting him through a simple prayer: 'Please God, let your life giving force flow into me and heal my mind and body'. Through faith, she believed this force to be flowing into her body, and gave thanks accordingly. As she observed the positive results she gained evidence of that which she had previously accepted on faith alone.

Sanford's thesis, that no matter how much we ask for something it becomes ours only as we accept it and give thanks for it, proved an inspiration for Evelyn. Her ideas had rekindled a faith Evelyn had relinquished, motivating her to experiment with her prayers. One approach had not produced the desired results, so she tried another. That, in fact, is the philosophy of this book. Any sort of prayer may not be to your taste, but perhaps you have not experimented with it, just as you may not have experimented with homoeopathic remedies or exercise. Until you try these avenues to healing you cannot tell whether they will help you or not.

INCREASING YOUR FAITH THROUGH COMBATING FEAR

Acting 'as-if' you possessed strong faith is one way of nurturing its growth. Another way is to combat the fear we have within us. As faith brings about that which we have faith in, so fear brings about the very things we fear.

Bob Montgomery is an intelligent, likeable man, but one who is constantly beset by fears. He always expects the worst, and by his very anticipation often makes unpleasant things happen. Many of our difficulties come to us because we believe they will come. Bob believes in the principle of hoping for the best but is unable to put it into practice. In reality, he is fearing the worst, knowing it is about to descend upon him. He tries to achieve an outward appearance of faith in his religion, that it will provide the comfort and support he craves, but he is really in the grasp of an inner fear. Acting 'as-if' he believes he will be healed does not work for Bob because he has an inner conviction that he is unable to tap a healing power. Thus, when he does try it is a most unconvincing attempt, one which he 'knows' is doomed to failure. Similarly he 'knows' doctors cannot help him when he is ill, nor can anyone else. His is a self-fulfilling prophecy which cuts him off from the healing power which is all around us. Faith and fear cannot exist together, for the latter engenders a doubt and foreboding, which negates the former.

To overcome his fear, Bob used imagery of the sort that has been mentioned frequently throughout this book. He would, in a relaxed state, visualize the situations which created fear within him and see himself handling them in the way he would like to. In addition, during the day he would use the 'windows in the mind' technique, letting unwanted fear-provoking thoughts float through. He came to realize he did not have to own all the thoughts which came into his mind. He could select only those which strengthened his faith, rejecting those which stimulated his fear.

Using the prayer of faith, Bob experimented with self-healing, being very careful to note any improvement. Any change for the better, even the slightest, provided cause for thanks. In the past, Bob had focussed on negatives, actually denying evidence of improvement in his health. Now he changed his focus, concentrating on positive signs.

Bob's improvement was gradually because he had to overcome a lifetime of fearful thinking. It is argued that everything that has ever happened to us is stored in our subconscious minds and that, by the time we are middle aged, most of us have accumulated a considerable store of doubts, fears, guilts and anxieties. Because these negative states influence the conscious mind, Bob, like most of us, had within him an inner self-destructive voice which continually undermined his faith. Despite his conscious efforts to reaffirm his belief in a healing power, he was plagued by his doubts and fears, expressed in terms of 'You don't really believe this will work do you? Maybe other people can be healed through faith but not you.' Bob carried out this re-education programme over a number of years so that the old habit of fearful thinking faded away through disuse to be replaced by a firm conviction that he could connect with and gain the healing power he sought.

It often seems as if there are several entities within us, pulling in different directions, and if we listen to our negative voices we become fearful of our own thoughts. But we do not have to listen to them and give them power over us. It all depends on where we choose to place our consciousness. If we think about our fears, seeing ourselves as being fearful, indecisive, limited, we have little hope of placing faith in the healing force that is there to be tapped. We can, however, place our consciousness in our positive belief, saying 'I believe in the availability of a healing power. I accept it. I feel it working within me. I am grateful for the healing that is at present occurring within me.'

This is not a matter of fighting your inner self-destructive entity but of turning your back on it, giving it no sustenance or support. It is a matter of letting go the old thought habits of fear and doubt, replacing them with new thought habits of faith and power. Imagine wiping the fearful thoughts from the blackboard of your mind, and deliberately thinking in terms of positive emotions. In this way you re-educate your subconscious mind, overcome your fears, and take off the fetters you have placed upon your faith.

THE HEALING OF BAD MEMORIES

Replacing negative emotions of fear, doubt, guilt and anxiety with positive ones of faith, love and joy has been stressed throughout this book. This is because it seems to be one of the most successful ways we know for improving our health. Partly this improvement of health stems from the healing power which can flow into us once we remove the barriers created by our negative emotions. In addition, there can be release from strain and anxiety if we choose to place our burdens upon a power greater than our own, but we must bear in mind that each of us chooses his or her own lifestyle and each must accept responsibility for his or her health, as pointed out in Chapters 2 and 13.

We have a need to be healed of bad memories for they exert a damaging influence upon our present existence. It is the concept of psychosomatic illness raising its head again, for the memories of past experiences can create illness and physical suffering unless we allow them to be healed. We can focus on a single event and expand it to fill our whole lives. All of us, I'm sure, know people who do this. Something unpleasant happens in their lives and it occupies their thoughts, their conversation, even their dreams, dominating their whole lives. This problem, and how to overcome it, is dealt with at length in *The Plus Factor*.

THE LAYING-ON OF HANDS

Faith plays a part, too, in healing through the laying-on of hands. This is a personal faith, that we have healing power within us. Some healers, including the famous Harry Edwards, felt his healing was due to spirit guides who worked through him. Whatever the mechanism involved, it does seem true that it is possible to influence a person's state of health by laying hands upon an injured part.

Some people have this power more strongly than others, but many who doubt their possession of this 'gift' have been amazed at their success in healing animals and promoting vigorous growth of diseased plants. When they turn to helping other people, they often find their curative powers increase with practice. But we need faith in ourselves, or in the forces which work through us, to make the initial attempts. Why not try yourself? You have nothing to lose.

This is what Mary Hawkins felt when her little girl was suffering considerable pain from a badly swollen, very tender big toe. Mary did not actually touch the area of inflammation, but gently stroked around it with a slow, circular motion. She never went beyond the border of tenderness. This sensitive area gradually contracted, becoming smaller and smaller until the inflammation disappeared. This slow approach linked with a stroking movement is often very successful.

Another equally successful technique is simply to lay your hand or hands lightly on the affected area. However, where extreme tenderness is present, it may be preferable to hold the hand or hands slightly above the skin so no actual contact is made. Should a joint be involved, such as the knee, the patient gradually increases the range of movement while the healer's hands are in position. The movement should never produce pain. Rather it explores the limits through which movement can take place before pain is experienced. As the healing continues this range of movement is extended until full use of the joint is restored. A number of treatment sessions may be necessary before this is achieved.

The use of 'the healing hand' seems to be very much an instinctive human reaction. It seems very natural for us to put our hand on a body part we have injured, perhaps rubbing or stroking as we do so. Yet it has been claimed that we are unable to heal ourselves in this way. Thought processes, suggestion, and the use of the imagination are seen to be effective methods of self-healing, but the laying on of hands cannot be successful because we are contacting our own auras. It is theorized that each of us is surrounded by an aura. Our bodies are energy systems such that when one part of our aura, that around our hand, enters another part of the same aura, that around our injured knee, energy is simply drawn from one part of the system to another. This, it is suggested, is insufficiently powerful to effect the restoration of damaged areas of the aura.

This view may have some validity but it seems to fly in the face of much common experience. We know that, quite frequently, we can ease pain by using our hands in the affected area. All you can do is experiment to find whether laying your hands on injured, painful parts of your body actually promotes healing. If it does, continue. If it does not, you might like to try imagination, 'seeing' a trusted friend or your imaginary doctor laying their hands upon your body, 'feeling' the healing energy flowing into you.

Headaches provide a complaint which often responds well to the laying on of hands. One of the more common treatments is to place the palms of the hands upon the area of pain (or an inch or two clear of the skin) and hold them there for several minutes. Then remove them, rub them together briskly for a moment or two, and replace them. Alternatively, gently stroking of the finger tips in one direction only, either downward or outward, is quite popular. By stroking away from the seat of the pain outwards, you will often feel the pain shifting as you move your fingertips so that as you draw your hands away from your head, the pain goes with them. Other hand movements you could use would be a clockwise, circular rubbing movement, or a fine, trembling vibratory movement of the fingers.

Healing headaches in this way does seem effective for many people. For others it is not. This is probably because some headaches are made worse by an increased flow of blood to the head, and such an increased flow is usually the result when hands are placed on an injury. Therefore, possibly the safest method is the gentle drawing of the fingers from the centre of the brow to the temples, thinking rhythmically 'peace-peace-peace' or 'calm-calm-calm'.

There are other circumstances, too, in which we would not wish to draw increased blood to a damaged area. The occurrence of a blood clot is obviously such a case. Here we can use the body forces centre. Lay one hand between the shoulder blades where the nerves of all organs are close to the body surface, and the other over the heart. A 'current' is usually felt to be passing between the hands, promoting general healing. The same technique can be used for any injury, one hand being placed on the seat of the pain and the other on the opposite side of the body. This is a treatment method particularly suited for the healing of others but there will be occasions you can use it to heal yourself.

Experiment to find which hand promotes more effective healing when placed on the painful area. In *The Rainbow in your Hands*, experimentalists Davis and Rawls suggest that it is the left hand which reduces pain and the right hand which strengthens weakened areas as long as no discomfort is present. However, you may find that this general conclusion is not true for you. Only experience will provide the answer.

Part 5
Natural Remedies

15. A Potpourri of Ideas

Previous chapters have outlined relatively systematic approaches to healing. However, many successful natural remedies exist which do not fit comfortably into any of these systems. This last chapter, then, will be somewhat different from earlier ones in that a number of different remedies, often having little relationship to each other, will be described.

WATER AS A HEALING AGENT

In a previous chapter, water, in the form of fomentations and ice, was mentioned as one means of stimulating acupressure points and reflexes. So valuable a healing agent is water that further elaboration is warranted.

Drinking pure water at body temperature is reputedly a great healing agent. Mineral water, too, is valuable, for the minerals occur in a natural balance. Large quantities of warm water help digestion and often stimulate a sluggish colon. Drinking a glass of warm or hot water, with a little lemon juice if desired, immediately on arising is a time tested remedy to flush out the system. No food is taken for at least twenty minutes after this early morning drink, which is said to eliminate toxins, stimulate circulation, calm the stomach, and encourage bowel action.

One of the best ways of taking water internally is in the form of herbal teas, which are easy to make, relatively pleasant to the taste, and often alleviate a wide range of symptoms. *Peppermint tea*, for example, may be used to combat chills, colic, dizziness, stomach flatulence, nausea, diarrhoea and influenza. Even nightmares are said to disappear if peppermint tea is taken before retiring. It is an excellent nighttime drink which cleanses and strengthens the body. *Sassafras tea*, too, is a cleanser of the entire body system, while *sage tea* makes an excellent tranquilizer, soothing the nerves, calming the digestion, and reducing flatulence.

Probably *valerian* is the best known 'nerve tonic' among the herbal teas. It is often used to promote sleep, but it also has pain relieving qualities. Another natural sedative is *camomille tea*. It, too, is of value to the insomniac, and, as well, relieves headaches and nervous tension generally. Where nausea is the problem, whether this is morning sickness, travel sickness or indigestion, *basil tea* is worth trying. It excels in promoting good digestion.

Rosemary tea serves a number of functions, but is particularly valuable for menstrual pains, nervous depression, colds and headaches. Should skin problems be in evidence, *lemon tea* is suggested as an acne reliever. Psoriasis, a skin complaint which is highly resistant to orthodox treatments, sometimes improves markedly if *sarsaparilla tea* is taken: fifteen grams is added to a litre of water and boiled for twenty minutes. Half of this amount is drunk while it is hot and the rest taken at intervals throughout the day.

Herbal teas have been used as a dietary aid, for they seem to act as appetite suppressants. If you are trying to lose weight, drink a glass of herbal tea about an hour before meals. You may find you require less food to satisfy your appetite. *Kelp* tablets achieve the same result, two being taken about an hour before meals.

There is a large range of herbal teas available, and it would be well worth your while to experiment with these, finding the ones which bring you health benefits. Most health stores carry large stocks together with literature on the particular uses to which each herb might be put. It is certainly an excellent way of enhancing the already great value of taking water internally.

In dealing with infection, the first 'medicine' should be pure water. This is taken internally for internal infections and externally for infected cuts and skin. Warm water is preferable because it increases metabolism and is more likely to draw out toxins and impurities from the body. Herbs such as *goldenseal, ginger, garlic* and *sassafras* help this process.

Water may be applied externally with great health benefits. Should you be sunburned, for example, the best treatment is to immediately bathe the skin in cold water for at least ten minutes. Burns, generally, are best handled in this way, being immediately immersed in cold water. Muscle strains and sprains, too, can be alleviated by the rapid application of cold water or, better still, ice packs, and their continuance for the next forty-eight hours. After this period, hot compresses are used. These may be alternated with cold compresses on a five minutes hot to one minute cold ratio.

Compresses or fomentations, which are thick pieces of cloth wrung out in hot or cold water, use the principle of moist heat or moist cold. Warm or hot fomentations provide natural relief for aching stiffness or pain in the internal organs and in the joints and muscles by stimulating the circulation. This increases the flow of nutrients to injured areas and promotes the removal of waste products. Pain in any part of the body indicates some form of congestion in the area affected, and alternating hot and cold fomentations will relieve this condition quicker than any other remedy. Compresses should be as hot as can be borne, to be followed either by a cold compress or a cold sponging.

Fomentations applied to either spine or abdomen help ease aching and stiff muscles generally, and low back pain in particular. The hot spinal pack, in which a thick piece of cloth is wrung out in hot water, placed on the spine and covered with a towel, soothes the nerve centres of the back so that spasm is relieved. The cold pack, in which the cloth is wrung out in cold water, stimulates and refreshes the nervous system. This same effect can be gained by a cold towel rub. The towel is wrung out in cold water and the arms, chest, abdomen, legs and back rubbed vigorously.

Warm moist heat can be generated by a shower, which may be used as an 'instrument' of zone therapy. The palms of the hands can be turned upwards so the needle point spray 'massages' them. If you are able to sit in the shower, raise the soles of your feet and let the needle spray 'massage' them too. Then turn your back so the water exerts pressure up and down your spine. This will relax the whole body, increase blood circulation and prove beneficial to nerve endings.

Though showers can thus promote a feeling of general well being, it is baths which are more popular as a healing water treatment. The hot bath, as hot as can be tolerated, relieves headaches, especially migraines for blood is drawn away from the brain. In addition, it helps the body relax, soothes nerves, calms the digestion, relieves pain in the joints and has a sedative effect. These baths should only be of short duration, for prolonged hot baths are not beneficial, having a stiffening effect on the body. If a stimulatory effect rather than a sedative effect is sought, finish with a cool or cold bath or shower by letting the cold water tap run.

Hot foot baths also exert a beneficial effect upon the system. Standing in a basin of ankle deep water for up to fifteen minutes at a time provides total body relaxation. It also does wonders for aching tired feet, particularly if the treatment is concluded by a one minute soak in cold water. Dry your feet well after the foot bath, probe for tender spots and massage them thoroughly. However, should the feet be bruised or injured, do not use the hot water treatment but cool them with ice cubes wrapped in a towel.

Epsom salts baths have a considerable reputation for treating sciatica, rheumatism and neuritis. Their effect is to aid the elimination of uric acid from the body. Approximately 1.3 kg of *Epsom salts* is added to half a tub of water which is as hot as can be comfortably tolerated. You remain in the bath until perspiring freely at which time you emerge, dry off, cover yourself with blankets, and gradually cool off.

Even haemorroids can benefit from water treatment. By sitting for half an hour a day in a warm bath, you relax the affected areas, permitting the body to naturally shrink the haemorroids.

Warm water, too, is helpful to the eyes. It is applied to the closed lids and is followed by the application of comfortably cool water. As our eyes are so important to us we will look at natural methods of treatment more closely.

THE TREATMENT OF THE EYES

Tired and swollen eyes can be soothed if a piece of cotton wool is soaked in cold water and placed over the closed eyelids. This treatment relaxes the eyes, and relaxation is really the key to improvement in eye function. Many visual defects are not organic in nature, but are the result of strain. Therefore, cure lies more in the elimination of this strain rather than in the use of glasses. Once you come to rely on the support given by your glasses, you accept your visual defects as part of you, as 'incurable'. This may be true in many cases but it is not always so.

Seeing in a relaxed way means letting things come to you rather than making an effort to see. Effort involves strain, and the tendency to stare becomes increasingly strong. Staring is completely unhelpful for it is an attempt to keep the eyes still, fixed rigidly on the object of attention. Yet, to see clearly, it is necessary to keep your eyes in motion. Should you be involved in close work which requires a concentrated gaze, it is advisable to occasionally look away at things in the distance. Let your eyes move around, changing their focus between the far distance and the close work upon which you are engaged. This applies, too, while you are driving. Do not stare, but let your eyes move about, focussing on objects which are differing distances from you. Frequent blinking should accompany such eye movement as it works against the staring tendency.

If your eyes are tired and itchy, do not rub them, but either soothe them with water or try 'palming'. Block out light by cupping your hands over your eyes without actually touching them. Think of the colour black. See only blackness. Imagine you are in a warm, dark, velvet lined room or are looking at a soft, black velvet curtain. Perhaps you are gazing out into deepest space where there is only pure blackness. Palm for periods of two or three minutes, or until your eyes feel more relaxed. As you remove your cupped hands and open your eyes, blink lightly and rapidly. Even if your eyes are not tired, it is worthwhile resting them in this way, or simply closing them when opportunity offers.

Tension in the muscles which control the eys can also be relieved. The eyes can be screwed up and the brows puckered to produce tension, then the tension is let go and the eyes relax. Other exercises involve movements of the eyeballs while the head is kept quite still. The eyeballs are moved in their sockets as far to the right as possible, then back to the left, then they look upwards and finally downwards. Stretch the movement to the limit for it is thought that by so doing you can increase the flexibility of the muscles controlling the eyes and possibly normalize your sight. That is, you may be able to overcome long- or short-sightedness if you practise regularly.

Other exercises to achieve the same end involve rotating the eyeballs clockwise and anti-clockwise. Changing focus from near to far distance has already been mentioned as a valuable sight improver. An exercise encouraging such shifting involves concentrating your gaze upon a finger tip held close to the eyes and then shifting away to focus on some object in the far distance. Repeating each of these exercises a number of times on a daily basis may lead to improvement of your sight. Trying them is the only way to find out.

Other ways of helping the eyes involve massage of the temples and neck to reduce fatigue, the use of a homoeopathic eye bath (two drops of *calendula* in cold water), increasing the intake of *Vitamin A* (carrots, sunflower seeds) to improve vision in poor light and increase tolerance to bright light, and introducing a drop of *castor oil* into the bloodshot eye.

Not only is *castor oil* a good remedy for bloodshot eyes, but it has been used most effectively to remove foreign bodies. Smear *castor oil* liberally under the eyelids. This provides a soothing film which tends to float the irritating material out of the eye.

Of course, *castor oil* is far more than an eye remedy. For centuries it has been used as a poultice, drawing inflammation, irritation and infection from the body through the skin. Usually the easiest way of making such a poultice is to warm 40-60 ml of *castor oil* to blood heat and spread it over the affected area. Then cover with a piece of old sheeting. The effect can be enhanced if the patient lies out in the warm sun, but, if this is impossible, he should lie quietly indoors for at least an hour. Poultices of this type will 'draw' abscesses, boils, carbuncles, splinters, insect stings and whitlows most effectively. Also, it has been suggested that *castor oil* used in this way will ease bronchial and chest infections generally.

Many people, in fact, see *castor oil* as something of a 'miracle' cure, using it as a general healing agent. As mentioned earlier in this book, introduced into each nostril, it has proven effective as a sinusitis cure when all else failed. At the other end of the body, massaging tired, bruised feet with warm *castor oil* and covering them with a pair of old cotton socks before going to bed produces wonderous relief by morning.

ENERGY AND VITALITY

Hopefully, the feeling of comfort in the feet thus engendered will make us more eager to get up in the morning. Many of us have a problem here, but not Barbara Jeffries. She believes a good day begins with her waking up procedure. As she drifts out of sleep, Barbara dreamily thinks of the coming day, visualizing things going well. She creates a positive expectancy for herself, a feeling of pleasant anticipation. When she first began thinking in this way, Barbara found it hard. For her, the waking up time was her low point for the day. Her thoughts were anything but optimistic. So she created a new habit, one which has changed her life in many ways, releasing an energy and vitality she did not know she possessed.

Vitality comes not only from the thoughts, however. Barbara does not jump straight out of bed. She spends time stretching every muscle in her body, languidly and fully. She turns her head slowly from side to side, up and down, so her neck rolls loosely. Her back arches, her legs stretch and she yawns widely. Stretching in this way gets the blood circulating and Barbara keeps it moving by, as she gets out of bed, shaking her legs, loosening up her knee and hip joints, and shaking her hands and wrists.

In the bathroom, she places her hands in a sink full of cold water. While doing so, she rolls a golf ball under each foot in turn. Keeping her spine straight, she inhales deeply through her nose and exhales through her mouth. She does this ten times. Time consuming? Not really. It takes only about five minutes, five minutes which charge Barbara with a level of energy that is the envy of her friends.

After a glass of warm water and lemon juice, she does ten minutes of stretching exercises. A beauty treatment, which involves putting ice water on her face and rubbing on the juice of a lemon, follows, and Barbara is then ready for breakfast. A terrible bore you might think. Obviously Barbara doesn't. She is now sixty-eight years old, looks fifteen years younger and possesses a vitality women twenty years her junior would envy. Perhaps she would be this way whatever she does. That is always possible, but she does not think so.

During the day, should she feel a lack of energy, Barbara snacks on a spoonful of peanut butter. As a variant she may stuff a stick of celery with peanut butter, or have a handful of cashew nuts or dates. These foods are good energy sources. In her diet, Barbara maximizes her intake of vitality-promoting magnesium and phosphorus rich foods. Kelp, wheat bran, wheatgerm, almonds, tomatoes and dandelion all figure prominently.

INSOMNIA

Though, many years ago she suffered from insomnia, Barbara has no such problem now. To some extent this may be due to her positive, unworried outlook on life, for much of our feeling of tiredness when we miss sleep is psychological. We expect to be tired next day because we know we have not had as much sleep as we 'should'. Yet, for most people, it is not really the lack of sleep which is the problem but the worry about this lack of sleep. Worry compounds itself really, for probably the main cause of insomnia is fretting about the difficulties of the day. Many 'instant cures' have been effected when people change their thoughts to create happiness and optimism.

A technique described in *The Plus Factor* suggests you remake your day as you rest in bed at night. Firstly think back over the good things which have happened. Feel cheerful about these. Then take the bad things one at a time, wiping them from the mind and remaking them, imagining them happening the way you would have preferred. This one simple technique has brought deep, refreshing sleep to many insomniacs.

Adopting a regular bedtime routine can help, also. Retire at the same time after the same set of non-stimulating evening activities. Exercise immediately before bedtime is not a good idea, nor is the intake of alcohol, coffee, tea, cola drinks and cigarettes. It is preferable to turn to natural sleep inducers such as a glass of warm *milk*, a slice of *cheese* or a piece of *chicken*. These are all rich in an amino acid called L-tryptophan which seems to exert a sedative effect.

Herbal teas can be useful in this context. *Valerian, catnip, lady's slipper, scullcap* and *hops* all may be of value in promoting sleep. Steep a teaspoonful in a cup of boiling water for ten minutes and drink it while hot. You will gain an added general tonic effect without the troublesome side effects of chemical sedatives. Should no herbs be available, try hot *grapefruit juice*.

Though naps during the day are generally beneficial, one taken after the evening meal is likely to make sleeping at night more of a problem. This problem may, however, be more imaginary than real for we do find it difficult to estimate how we have spent the night. People who complain about sleeping little usually wildly underestimate the length of time they have slept. Laboratory experiments have revealed this repeatedly. Subjects claim they have been awake all night, yet monitoring devices reveal they may have slept anything from four to eight hours. Perhaps we sleep too much anyway. Thomas Edison is quoted as saying: 'Most people overeat 100 per cent and oversleep 100 per cent because they like it. That extra 100 percent makes them unhealthy and inefficient.'

IONIZATION OF THE AIR

Something else that makes us unhealthy and inefficient may be the very air we breathe. The air around us normally contains millions of electrically charged particles called ions which have a stimulating effect on body activity. As air passes through sunlight and over water it takes on this slight electrical charge. When air charged in this way comes into contact with airborne pollutants, it discharges onto them, drawing them harmlessly to earth. Thus the air is kept pollutant-free and fresh smelling. This process continues as long as the ionized air is produced faster than the pollutants.

In cities, this is not the case. Tons of pollutants are dumped into the air every day, destroying the natural balance. Because the cleansing ions are used at a rate faster than they can be produced, the air becomes stale and dirty. Within the household, too, the same process takes place. Cigarette smoke, cooking odours and dust foul the air. Central heating and air conditioning compound the problem, stripping the air of its cleansing ions. This depletion leads to respiratory troubles, general discomfort, lethargy, and loss of physical and mental efficiency. It has been estimated that approximately 70 per cent of the population is likely to be adversely affected by polluted air in one or more of these ways.

In a dry, centrally heated room we are likely to feel stuffy, depressed and irritable, somewhat the same as we would feel before a storm. This is due to the preponderance of positive ions in the air. However, after a storm, we usually feel a sense of exhilaration. The same euphoric feeling can also be experienced near moving water, such as surf or waterfalls, or on mountain tops. In these cases, there is a preponderance of negative ions in the air. Generators are available which duplicate this effect, through releasing a stream of negative ions into the atmosphere.

Negative ion generators have been used in European hospitals where, it is claimed, they have eliminated or drastically reduced postoperative pain and speeded up recovery time. Burn units, particularly, have reported accelerated healing if negative ion generators are placed in rooms where patients are being treated. Experimental work conducted in offices and factories suggest that the improved atmospheric conditions lead to a general reduction in tension and in respiratory problems. Absenteeism, due to sickness, declines markedly.

These generators are available commercially and private users have reportedly derived considerable benefit from them. Mainly these reports focus on greatly reduced incidence of respiratory problems such as sinusitis, bronchitis, hay fever and asthma. However, there is also evidence of improved ability to concentrate for long periods of time. The drowsiness and sleepiness which usually overtakes us when we study or read intensively in a closed room, seems to be held in abeyance. Mental efficiency is thus enhanced.

Apart from using a negative ion generator in your room, there are other things you can do to shake off lethargy, and to clear stuffy heads and blocked sinuses. Keep windows open as much as possible, sit beside water, particularly moving water, whenever you can, breathe fresh country air and climb to the top of hills occasionally. When you walk, try to do so away from air-polluted areas. Breathe deeply as you walk, practicing the rhythmic methods outlined in an earlier chapter. Being aware of the value of negatively charged air may, in itself, help you considerably, for you will be more likely to seek such environments. For more information on this subject, read *The Ion Effect* by Fred Soyka.

LONGEVITY AND STRESS

By doing so, you are likely to reduce your stress level. Sitting quietly beside water, breathing fresh air, and climbing hills or mountains are activities which relax both mind and body. Reduction of stress is emerging increasingly as one of the factors promoting longevity, together with systematic under-eating, periodic fasting, exercise, regular habits and a positive attitude of living each day to the full. Throughout this book are scattered many ways through which you might achieve this stress reduction, all of which are probably better than the remedy adopted by most people—chemical tranquilizers.

Many natural tranquilizers exist which produce comparable

results and do so without the unwanted side effects. One of these is the herbal remedy, *pacifenity*, a tablet which contains *passiflora*, *mistletoe*, *avena sativa*, *valerian*, *gentian*, *hops*, *scullcap* and *motherwort*. *Valerian*, alone, as a homoeopathic remedy, is an effective tranquilizer, as are the others, such as *Argentum nitricium* and *Kali Phos.*, mentioned in the chapters on homoeopathy. Vitamin B_6, too, would seem to have claims as a natural tranquilizer.

When under stress, you would be well advised to make use of another natural substance, Vitamin C. Tension deprives the adrenals of their store of this vitamin within seconds and it is necessary to replace it as soon as possible. Such Vitamin C depletion might be one reason why people under constant stress fall ill, for Vitamin C is a great infection fighter and its lack in the body weakens our resistance to disease.

Perhaps the best stress reliever of all though is something we have within us, the gift of laughter. Norman Cousins, referred to in the first chapter, is living proof of its value as a curative agent, and it would certainly appear to be one of the secrets of longevity. Laughter can express many things not immediately apparent, channelling off feeling such as repressed anger, embarrassment, and anxiety. We could all probably do with a sense of the ridiculous so that we can laugh not only at others but also at ourselves. It is not easy to do this for we are so often puffed up with vanity, so conscious of our importance, that we take ourselves too seriously. However, once we can stand off and watch ourselves posturing and pretending to be something we are not, it becomes easier to laugh at our own foibles.

Laughter helps us cope with stress. It provides a sort of safety valve when the pressure builds up so that we turn the harsh realities of life into jokes. The television series M*A*S*H, and the film of the same name on which it was based, is an excellent example of this. Doctors working on soldiers wounded during warfare would find it difficult to cope with the daily procession of shattered bodies without humour as a saviour.

Work, too, seems to play its part in contributing to longevity. Studies on the peasant peoples of the USSR and of Eastern Europe confirm that people who keep working live longer, and do so in good health. Retirement, in Western society, is fast becomming a major health hazard. Not for all, of course. Many people thrive on retirement, but usually because they keep active and occupied. So perhaps it is not work per se that promotes longevity. Rather it is the fact it provides an activity which keeps people busy.

ARTHRITIS

Work, however, does not seem to provide a cure for arthritis. Still, if you are afflicted with this ailment there are several natural remedies which may bring you the relief you seek. One of these is to soak four *dried apricots* overnight in water. In the morning drink the water and eat the apricots three-quarters of an hour before eating breakfast. Another remedy is to take *vegetable tablets*, available at health stores, with your meals. A third is, at mealtimes, to sip a mixture of 10 ml of *apple cider vinegar* and two teaspoons of *honey* in water. Fourth, try the external treatment of filling a basin with water, adding 2 tablespoons of *Epsom salts*, and bathing in it. Alternate hot and cold baths in which your hands and feet are immersed twice a day is another water treatment likely to provide relief. Dipping a towel in hot water and wrapping it around the aching joints may help, too.

These remedies are palliatives. Perhaps, the real cure for arthritis lies in the mind rather than in the body. Dorothy Hall, in *The Natural Health Book*, said: 'I have never had an arthritic patient who was not a person who suppressed his angers and frustrations and stresses, went bravely on doing his duty and never let the side down'. This burying of acid emotional reactions Hall sees as complicating an acid condition of body tissues. If she is correct in diagnosing arthritis as a psychosomatic illness, the natural emotional release of stress and strain should contribute to a healing of the condition.

Choice of appropriate foods should make a positive condition, too. Foods high in sodium such as *whey, kelp, olives, celery* and *horseradish* are valuable as they help preserve suppleness and ease of movement. Potassium-rich foods, *tomatoes*, *kelp*, *dried fruits*, *potatoes*, *parsley*, *sunflower seeds*, *horseradish* and *legumes*, play an important part, also, for their action is that of reducing the level of uric acid in the blood. *Red cherries* and *strawberries*, taken on an empty stomach between meals, are particularly effective in achieving this result. Food which produces uric acid such as meat, eggs, fish, milk, salt and peas should be eaten sparingly.

VITAMIN C

As is the case with so many ailments, *Vitamin C*, first brought to public awareness by Nobel Prize winner Linus Pauling, has a part to play in the relief of arthritis. *Calcium*, though it may seem almost contradictory to say so, can be helpful in many cases of arthritis. However, to avoid the danger that it may be deposited in the joints and so exacerbate the problem, a high potency *Vitamin C* tablet is taken with the *calcium* tablet. But, of course, the uses of *Vitamin C* go far beyond this.

It may be used to alleviate the bruising, both internal and external, which usually results from surgery or accidental injury. In this respect it plays a similar role to the homoeopathic remedies, *Arnica* and *Bellis*. If taken for several weeks before entering hospital, *Vitamin C* helps strengthen the tissues against the shock of the operation. Continuance of dosage after surgery will facilitate a rapid, infection free recovery.

As mentioned earlier, it is preferable to take *Vitamin C* in its natural form though, where large doses are required, synthetic supplements become necessary. As a daily routine, a cup of *rosehip tea*, perhaps sweetened with honey, will provide a suitable amount. However, should you be under considerable stress, be taking cortisone, antibiotics or sulpha drugs, or be a smoker, it is necessary to increase your *Vitamin C* intake. The body can absorb large amounts of *Vitamin C* without harm, that which is not required being secreted in the urine.

Vitamin C, in an amount of up to ten grams a day, can be taken if your body is exposed to a heavy dosage of drugs. It exerts an anti-toxic effect, as does lecithin which may also be taken to offset the effects of drugs on the body. Two or three tablespoons of lecithin a day are necessary to achieve this result. *Vitamin B complex*, either in the form of high potency tablets or in natural form as yoghurt and whey should be taken when antibiotics are prescribed, and continued after this drug treatment ceases in order to re-establish new flora of beneficial bacteria.

Sinus infections often yield to *Vitamin C*. However, the chances of a 'cure' are enhanced if garlic-horseradish tablets are taken as well. *Vitamin B_6* could provide a third curative agent. The combination of *Vitamin C* and *garlic* is possibly the best natural treatment available for all types of colds, sore throats, and respiratory troubles. With a throat infection, it is helpful to keep a clove of *garlic* or a *Vitamin C* tablet in the mouth, held between the cheek and teeth.

Earlier it was mentioned that *Vitamin C* may be taken with calcium to prevent the latter being deposited in the joints. It may also be taken with aspirin. This increases the effectiveness of the aspirin, making it work longer and harder. Incidentally, it is advisable to take aspirin crushed, dissolved in water, or chewed with a mouthful of milk to minimize stomach irritation.

Should you be troubled by allergies, it would be worthwhile taking large doses of *Vitamin C*. Apparently, among its many virtues, this vitamin acts as a natural antihistamine. An amount of between two and five grams daily, divided into several doses, would be sufficient to demonstrate whether this form of treatment will relieve your allergies.

MUSCLE AND LEG PROBLEMS

After unaccustomed exercise or heavy work, our muscles become quite stiff. Large doses of *Vitamin C* may be used both for prevention and treatment. The homoeopathic remedies of *Arnica* and *Bellis* perform the same function. As a treatment method, alternate hot and cold compresses can be very beneficial.

Where muscle and joint soreness is a more constant problem, 5 ml of *cod liver oil* taken at least twice a week may provide relief. An external application of *wheat germ oil* has also produced excellent results where muscles are stiff or sore.

It is often with our legs that we suffer most. To keep our legs in better health, one simple thing to do is avoid crossing them. When we cross our legs we put additional strain on our sacroilliac, and contribute to the development of varicose veins. Should you already have this problem, each day practise the yogic shoulder stand posture. Also elevate the foot of your bed 8-10 cm. Avoid sitting whenever possible, for this is seen as a major cause of varicose veins. Instead, walk, swim, or cycle as much as you can. Long periods of standing are also to be avoided.

Should cramping in the legs be your problem, there are a number of avenues you may care to explore. Leg and joint stretching exercises, as outlined in the exercise chapter, are likely to increase suppleness and flexibility. This is a gradual process, however, and naturally, you would wish for quicker relief. *Calcium lactate*, taken in tandem with *Vitamin C*, is a well tried remedy. So, too, is *magnesium*. A third possibility is *Vitamin E*; 400 to 500 IUs (international units) taken daily has proven effective in a number of cases.

DIGESTIVE PROBLEMS

Several of the natural remedies already mentioned are of particular interest to those who suffer from stomach complaints. Beth Parsons is such a person. All of us seem to have one particular weak area in our system. With some, it is with the throat, with others the chest. Beth's weak spot is her stomach. Whenever anything goes wrong with her health, her stomach is sure to be involved.

Flatulence used to be an almost constant companion. Most meals were followed by a distended stomach and a lot of gas. Medical examination had revealed no physical abnormality and the tablets prescribed provided little relief. Actually, Beth found her own solution in a book of household remedies. Should she feel 'gassy', she lies down on her face, rolls on to her left side, and on to her right side. She then gets to her feet and drinks a cup of hot water. If this procedure does not solve the problem, she lies down in such a way that her anus is higher than her head. Should this fail, too, she eats a clove of *garlic* which is really the supreme remedy. It neutralizes the putrefactive toxins and kills undesirable bacteria, thus eliminating gas and also relieving indigestion.

Actually, Beth would prefer to use *garlic* as her first treatment but her family rather object to the odour. Out of deference to their sensitivity, she tries the other approaches first. Should she need to take *garlic*, she eats a sprig or two of *parsley* or chews on a *coffee bean* afterwards to somewhat sweeten her breath.

It is just as well Beth has found ways of handling the 'garlic breath' for she has found this herb to be an excellent diarrhoea preventative. Before discovering her 'magic remedy', she suffered bouts of diarrhoea several times a year. Should she, for one reason or another, cease taking *garlic* on a regular basis, then the attacks return. To treat them, she first uses natural methods. Non-bacterial chronic diarrhoea is usually relieved very quickly by three tablespoons of *raw unprocessed wheat bran* in fruit juice. *Yoghurt* is another possible treatment, though acidophilus culture works faster. Even something as simple as 10 ml of *apple cider vinegar* has been a successful diarrhoea remedy for some people.

Some experts would suggest tea and toast as the best diet for a diarrhoea sufferer. They suggest the avoidance of solid foods but the drinking of a lot of fluid in the form of water and weak teas. Milk and all dairy products should be avoided, together with raw vegetables, fried foods, raw fruits, bran, spices and coffee. It is interesting that bran is included in this list, for Beth has found this to be a most effective treatment agent. This contradiction only serves to confirm the basic theme of this book. Though expert opinion can serve as a guide, you must be your own 'expert' and that means you must try out things for yourself.

Constipation, the opposite side of the coin, also requires the drinking of a lot of fluid, possibly double or treble your normal intake. The key element in treatment lies in the introduction of considerable bulk into the diet. *Raw vegetables*, salads, bran, raw fruit, prunes and dates provide such bulk. *Yoghurt* and acidophilus culture, mentioned in the treatment of diarrhoea, also are useful in cases of constipation. This is because they function as bowel regulators. *Honey* and *garlic* do, too. Even *Vitamin C*, that ubiquitous remedy, can help the constipation sufferer. One to three grams a day is the suggested dosage.

Figs are an excellent remedy for constipation. In fact, this fruit has a wide range of healing uses. If the fruit is broken off from the tree before it is ripe, a milk escapes which may be used to treat sores, boils and warts. A warm tea made from the leaves is helpful if applied externally to bruises, and spots on the face and body. Taken internally, the tea has a curative effect on diseased lungs. It also soothes sore throats and can be quite effective in relieving earache.

A final natural constipation remedy is *slippery elm* which is available in tablet form. A bowel cleanser-regulator, this remedy is excellent for all bowel and bladder problems, stomach and kidney troubles, boils and inflammations, bronchitis, ulcerated stomach and fever. It can be of assistance in relieving the discomfort of stomach ache, but probably *raw sauerkraut juice, peppermint tea* or *camomille tea* would be more successful in dealing with this problem.

A FINAL WORD

Within the pages of this book I have described many natural remedies which have stood the test of time. I have tried to abstract these from a vast literature derived from many centuries of usage. It is unavoidable that the choices I have made reflect my own experience and my own biases. Many excellent approaches to healing have, no doubt, been overlooked. However, no one book could hope to encompass all the wisdom of natural healing. The books to which I have referred provide avenues for you to pursue particular healing approaches further should you wish to do so.

In conclusion, I would like to restate a point made at the beginning of the book. Natural or 'unorthodox' medicine is not all virtuous. Nor is 'orthodox' medicine. Both are valuable and

A Potpourri of Ideas 261

should be used where appropriate. However, as natural remedies normally do no harm, producing no dangerous side effects, they are preferable as a first line of treatment. Except in real emergencies, experiment to see whether you can heal your ailment naturally. If you cannot, then drugs and surgery are the next steps.

This is what taking personal responsibility for your health is all about. Unless you take steps to find out what forms of treatment can help you, you are left with no choice but to use orthodox medicine. Although it can help you in many ways, it is a far from perfect system of health care. Even its staunchest adherents would admit that. Therefore you have room for manoeuvre, to be your own 'expert', and learn how best to heal your own body. It is an exciting and rewarding activity, one which I hope brings you both health and happiness.

Bibliography

P. AIROLA, *How to Get Well*, Health Plus Publishers, Phoenix, 1974.

E. BACH, *The Twelve Healers and Other Remedies*, Daniel & Co., London, 1952.

A. BERGSON AND V. TUCHACK, *Zone Therapy*, Pinnacle, New York, 1974.

M. BLACKIE, *The Patient Not the Cure*, Woodbridge Press, Santa Barbara, 1978.

M. BLATE, *The Natural Healers Acupressure Handbook*, Routledge and Kegan Paul, London, 1978.

W. BOERICKE, *Homoeopathic Materia Medica* (9th edit.), Boericke and Runyon, Philadelphia, 1927.

G. BRODSKY, *From Eden to Aquarius*, Bantam, New York, 1974.

J. V. CERNEY, *Handbook of Unusual and Unorthodox Healing Methods*, Parker, New York, 1976.

P. M. CHANCELLOR, *Handbook of the Bach Flower Remedies*, Daniel and Co., Essex, 1971.

E. CHERASKIN, W. M. RINGSDORF, JR and A. BRECHER, *Psychodietetics*, Bantam, New York, 1974.

N. COUSINS, 'Anatomy of an Illness (As Seen by a Patient)', *Journal of Holistic Health*, 4, 94-101, 1979.

A. R. DAVIS and W. C. RAWLS, JR, *The Rainbow in Your Hands*, Exposition Press, New York, 1976.

J. DIAMOND, *Your Body Doesn't Lie*, Harper and Row, Sydney, 1979.

E. FINCH and B. FINCH, *The Pendulum and Your Health*, Esoteric Publications, Sedona, Arizona, 1977.

J. GRAEDON, *The People's Pharmacy*, St Martin's Press, New York, 1976.

T. GRAVES, *Dowsing*, Turnstone, London, 1976.

D. HALL, *The Natural Health Book*, Nelson, Melbourne, 1976.

Bibliography

I. ILLICH, *Medical Nemesis,* Pantheon Books, New York, 1976.

B. JENCKS, *Respiration for Relaxation, Invigoration and Special Accomplishment,* Jencks, Utah, 1974.

J. KINGSTON, *Healing Without Medicine,* Aldus Books, London, 1976.

A. MALLESON, *Need Your Doctor Be Useless?,* Allen and Unwin, London, 1973.

L. MOREHOUSE AND L. GROSS, *Total Fitness,* Mayflower, St Albans, Herts, 1977.

D. NORFOLK, *The Habits of Health,* St Martin's Press, New York, 1976.

V. OBECK AND R. AITKIN, *The Complete Book of Isometrics,* Beaverbrook Newspapers, London, 1978.

I. OYLE, *The Healing Mind,* Celestial Arts, Millbrae, California, 1975.

E. W. RUSSELL, *Report on Radionics,* Spearman, London, 1973.

M. SAMUELS and H. BENNETT, *The Well Body Book,* Bookworks/Random House, New York, 1973.

A. SANFORD, *The Healing Light,* Logos, Plainfield, New Jersey, 1972.

K. SCHNERT, *How to Be Your Own Doctor (Sometimes),* Grosset and Dunlap, New York, 1975.

H. SELYE, *Stress Without Distress,* J. B. Lippincott, Philadelphia, 1974.

C. N. SHEALY, *Occult Medicine,* Dial Press, New York, 1975.

I. SHERMAN, *Natural Remedies,* Naturegraph, Healdsburg, Calif., 1970.

W. E. SHUTE with H. J. TAUB, *Vitamin E for Ailing and Healthy Hearts,* Pyramid Books, New York, 1972.

F. SOYKA with A. EDMONDS, *The Ion Effect,* Bantam, New York, 1978.

H. E. STANTON, *The Plus Factor: a guide to positive living,* Fontana/Collins, Sydney, 1979.

J. H. STEPHENSON, *A Doctor's Guide to Helping Yourself with Homoeopathic Remedies,* Parker, New York, 1976.

A. WIGMORE, *Be Your Own Doctor,* Dan Pilla, St Paul, undated.

Index

Aches
  cell salt remedies 91
  homoeopathic remedies 48, 57
  muscle problems 257-8
  relief through imagination 198
  water treatment 245
Allergies 257
Aluminium cooking utensils 31
  dowsing for harmful effects 110
Anaemia 89
Animals 85
Antibiotic, vegetable 154
Arm problems 123, 125
Arthritis (*see also* Uric Acid,
  Gout) 255-6
  cell salt remedy 91
  fasting 165
Ask-the-doctor list 36
Aspirin 257
Asthma
  cell salt remedies 90
  fasting 165
  homoeopathic remedies 63
  negative ion generator
    treatment 252
  vegetable juice treatment 157

Back problems
  acupressure point treatment
    123-4
  cell salt remedies 90
  exercise treatment 174
  homoeopathic remedies 44
  imagination exercise 199
  reflexology treatment 139
  water treatment 245
Babies 85
Bed-wetting 51
Black eye 60
Bladder problems 89
Bleeding
  homoeopathic remedy 58
  nose 58
Blood clots 90
Blood pressure, lowering
  cell salt remedies 92
  garlic 155
Body cleanser 156
Body signals 33-4
Boils 46
Bone injuries
  cell salt remedies 88
  homoeopathic remedies 69
Bronchial problems
  castor oil poultice 249
  cell salt remedies 89
  garlic 155
Bruising
  homoeopathic remedies 56-7
  vitamin C treatment 256
Burns
  homoeopathic remedies 56, 59
  mouth 58
  negative ion generator
    treatment 252
  slow healing 59
  water treatment 245

Carbuncles 46
Cancer 206
Castor oil, uses for
  eyes 248
  sinus infection 15
Childbirth 85
Children 85
Chilblains
  exercise treatment 174
  homoeopathic remedies 62
Chills
  herbal teas 243
  homoeopathic remedies 56
Cod liver oil 149
Coffee 152
Colds
  acupressure point treatment 123-5
  breathing exercise 197
  cell salt remedies 89
  fruit juice treatment 157
  garlic 155
  herbal teas 244
  homoeopathic remedies 54, 63, 66, 68
  honey 155
  reflexology treatment 128, 139
  vitamin C treatment 74
Confidence, lack of 76
Constipation 259-60
  fasting 165
  homoeopathic remedies 45
  nutritional treatment 154-5
  water treatment 243
Corns 58
Coughs
  acupressure point treatment 123-5
  breathing exercise 197
  homoeopathic remedies 51
Cousins, Norman 20
Cramps
  cell salt treatment 91
  reflexology treatment 140
Cuts 56

Decision making 100-1
Depression
  Bach remedies 78
  homoeopathic remedies 67
Diarrhoea
  acupressure point treatment 124-5
  herbal teas 243
  homoeopathic remedies 51, 64
  nutritional treatment 259
Doctor, imaginary 39-41
Drowsiness
  homoeopathic remedies 61
  negative ion generator treatment 252
Drugs
  dangers 20-4
  offset their effects 256

Ear problems
  acupressure point treatment 123, 126
  reflexology treatment 128, 139-40
Emergency treatment
  Bach remedies 76
  homoeopathic remedies 56-7
Energizer, natural 157
Energy 249-50
  breathing exercises 191-3
Eye problems 247-9
  acupressure point treatment 126
  breathing exercise 197
  eyewash 58
  reflexology treatment 128, 140
  water treatment 246-7

Fatigue
  acupressure point treatment 124
  Bach remedies 76, 78
  homoeopathic remedies 58
  ice packs 129
Fear
  Bach remedies 76, 78
  homoeopathic remedies 51, 64
  imagery treatment 234

Feet, tired
  castor oil treatment 249
  water treatment 246
Females, problems specific to
  acupressure point treatment 125
  garlic 155
  herbal teas 241
  homoeopathic remedies 66
  vegetable juice treatment 157
Food poisoning 46

Garlic 155
Germ-theory of disease 25-6
Gout (*see also* Uric acid, Arthritis)
  cell salt remedies 91-2
  homoeopathic remedies 59
  vegetable juice treatment 157
Grief 52, 68

Habits
  changing 27-8, 30
  of health 25, 27-8
Haemorroids
  acupressure point treatment 123
  cell salt remedies 88
  reflexology treatment 140
  water treatment 246
Hang-over remedies 60
Hay fever
  fasting 165
  homoeopathic remedies 63
  negative ion generator
    treatment 253
  reflexology treatment 139
  vegetable juice treatment 157
Headaches
  acupressure point treatment
    123-4, 126
  Bach remedies 73
  cell salt remedies 89
  herbal teas 244
  homoeopathic remedies 61
  imagination healing 198
  jogging 172
  touch healing 153

  suggestion healing 210-11
  water treatment 246
Heat exhaustion 63
Herbal teas 243-4
Hiccoughs 140
Hip problems 128
Hives 51, 59
Holistic health
  body harmony 34
  definition 19

Indecisiveness 76, 79
Indigestion
  cell salt remedies 92
  homoeopathic remedies 51
Infection
  cell salt remedies 92
  fruit juice treatment 157
  garlic 155
  honey 155
  reflexology treatment 140
  water treatment 244-5
Inflammation
  castor oil poultice 248
  cell salt remedies 89
  touch healing 237
Influenza
  acupressure point treatment 124
  herbal teas 243
  homoeopathic remedies 52-3, 62
Insomnia 34, 250-1
  herbal teas 244
  homoeopathic remedies 60-1, 67
  honey 156
  self-hypnosis 216
  separation from 222
  vegetable juice treatment 157
Irritability
  Bach remedies 75, 78
  homoeopathic remedies 45, 51
Itching 198

Jealousy 73
Jogging 30
Jung, Carl 29

Kelp 149
Kidney stones 70

Leg problems
  acupressure point treatment
    123-4
  cell salt remedies 88
Life force 25
Lifestyle 27-8
Longevity 253-5
  and exercise 176-7, 180
  fasting 165

Materia Medica 50-2, 108
Meditation 30
Memory, weak 61
Mental centering 195
Migraine
  acupressure point treatment 126
  homoeopathic remedies 68-9

Napping 221
Nerves (*see also* Stress, Tension)
  cell salt remedies 90
  herbal teas 244
  homoeopathic remedies 61, 63
  reflexology treatment 138
  vegetable juice treatment 157
  water treatment 246
Nettlerash 59
Nightmares 244
Nuts 154

Pain relief
  acupressure point treatment 123, 126-7
  herbal teas 244
  homoeopathic remedies 68
  imagination exercises 223-4
  laying-on of hands 237-9
  mind as amplifier 222-3
  water treatment 245-6
Parsley 153
Patient-doctor relationship 35-9
Placebo
  definition 48
  positive attitude, and 20, 208-9
  suggestion, and 212
  trust in doctor 37
Potatoes 154
Plants
  Bach remedies 85
  dowsing their needs 111
Prayer of faith 231-3
Prostrate problems 157
Psychosomatic illness 228-30

Resentment 68
Rheumatism
  cell salt remedies 89, 91
  homoeopathic remedies 56
  vegetable juice treatment 157
Ringworm 62
Rose hips 149

Sciatica 157
Self-hypnosis
  induction 213-5
  split-screen healing technique 215
Self-pity 78
Sex, and exercise 178
Sexual problems 67
Shingles 64
Shock
  Bach remedies 76
  homoeopathic remedies 56
  vitamin C treatment 256
Shoulder injury 128
Simonton, Carl 206
Sinus trouble
  acupressure point treatment 126
  breathing exercise 197
  castor oil treatment 15
  chlorophyll 156
  garlic 155
  garlic and horseradish 257
  homoeopathic remedies 63
  negative ion generator treatment 253
  reflexology treatment 139
  vegetable juice treatment 156

Skin problems
   acupressure point treatment 123
   Bach remedies 79
   cell salt remedies 89-90, 92
   fasting 165
   garlic 155
   herbal teas 244
   homoeopathic remedies 56, 62
   vegetable juice treatment 156
Spasms 91
Sports injuries
   cell salt remedies 89, 93
   homoeopathic remedies 57, 66, 69
Stings 59
Stomach problems 258-9
   acupressure point treatment 124-5
   breathing exercise 199
   cell salt remedies 89
   fruit juice treatment 157
   garlic 155
   herbal teas 243-4
   homoeopathic remedies 46, 50-1, 56, 62, 64, 69
   honey 156
   reflexology treatment 131
   self-diagnosis 148
   yoghurt 155
Stress (*see also* Nerves, Tension) 253-5
   action meditation 220
   body's self-defence reaction 29
   breathing, and 39
   caused internally 218
   daily relaxation session 194-6
   exercise, and 178, 218
   herbal remedy 254
   laughter, and 254
   mantra 220
   reflexology treatment 138
   relaxation tape 221
   relief through imagination 221-2
   test of stress level 217
   vitamin C treatment 254

Sunburn 244
Swimming 174

Teething troubles 51
Tension (*see also* Nerves, Stress)
   Bach remedies 76
   homoeopathic remedies 45
Tetanus 60
Throat, sore
   acupressure point treatment 123, 126
   breathing exercise 197
   cell salt remedies 89
   fruit juice treatment 157
   homoeopathic treatment 70
   reflexology treatment 139
Toothache
   acupressure point treatment 123
   reflexology treatment 128
Travel sickness
   acupressure point treatment 124-5
   herbal teas 244
   homoeopathic remedies 58, 62

Ulcers 165
Uric acid, elemination (*see also* Arthritis, Gout)
   epsom salt bath 246
   nutritional treatment 153-4, 256
Urticaria 46

Vaccination, ill effects of 69
Varicose veins 174
Vitamin C 256-7
   cold preventative 74
   combine natural and synthetic 150
   dowsing for needs 115-17
   for self-healing 21
   stress, and 254
Voice, loss of 59
   acupressure point treatment 126

Walking 173
Warts 69, 212

Weight control 129-69
  dowsing to select weight loss plan 118
  exercise, and 174
  herbal teas 244
  kelp tablets 244
  through mind control 224
Whey powder 149
Wounds
  cell salt remedies 89
  homoeopathic remedies 58, 60

Yeast 149
  as appetite suppressant 164

About the Author

After graduating from Melbourne University, Harry Stanton spent eight years teaching in secondary schools and five years lecturing in teachers' colleges. Since 1969 he has taught in the universities of South Australia and Tasmania. At present he is Consultant on Higher Education at the University of Tasmania. In addition, he provides a consultancy service for companies and the public sector as well as conducting a private practice in clinical and sports psychology.

He is the author of three other Optima books:
THE PLUS FACTOR: *A Guide to Positive Health* (February 1988)
THE STRESS FACTOR: *A Guide To More Relaxed Living* (August 1988)
THE FANTASY FACTOR: *Using Your Imagination To Solve Everyday Problems* (August 1988)